The New England Healthcare Assembly

Managing Patient
Expectations

. . . .

Susan Keane Baker

Managing Patient Expectations

The Art of Finding and
Keeping Loyal Patients

Jossey-Bass Publishers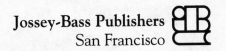
San Francisco

The quote from Jackie Robinson on p. 1 is used by permission of TM/© 1997 Rachel Robinson under license authorized by CMG Worldwide, Inc., Indianapolis, Indiana, 46256 USA. The quote from Norm Brodsky on p. 71 is reprinted with permission of *Inc.* magazine. Goldhirsh Group, Inc., 38 Commercial Wharf, Boston, Ma. 02110. *Listen and Earn*, Norm Brodsky, March 1997, p. 33 (http://www.inc.com). Reproduced by permission of the publisher via Copyright Clearance Center, Inc.

Jossey-Bass books and products are available through most bookstores. To contact Jossey-Bass directly, call (888) 378–2537, fax to (800) 605–2665, or visit our website at www.josseybass.com.

Substantial discounts on bulk quantities of Jossey-Bass books are available to corporations, professional associations, and other organizations. For details and discount information, contact the special sales department at Jossey-Bass.

 Manufactured in the United States of America on Lyons Falls Turin Book. This paper is acid-free and 100 percent totally chlorine-free.

Library of Congress Cataloging-in-Publication Data

Baker, Susan Keane.
    Managing patient expectations / the art of finding and keeping
loyal patients / by Susan Keane Baker.
        p.   cm.
    Includes bibliographical references and index.
    ISBN 0-7879-4158-1 (hc. : alk. paper)
    1. Patient satisfaction.   2. Physician and patient.   3. Ambulatory
medical care.   4. Consumer satisfaction.   I. Title.
    [DNLM: 1. Patient Satisfaction.   2. Outpatients—psychology.
3. Knowledge, Attitudes, Practice.   4. Patient Participation.
5. Physician-Patient Relations.   W 85 B168m 1998]
R727.3.B28   1998
610.69'6—dc21
DNLM/DLC
for Library of Congress   98-15900

FIRST EDITION
HB Printing   10 9 8 7 6 5 4 3 2

Contents

Part Four: Responding to Unmet Expectations

Part Five: Exceeding Expectations

Preface

Satisfied patients are the key to professional success and the personal rewards of medicine. Every physician prefers loyal patients who are satisfied with the care they receive. When a patient is not satisfied, he may seek care elsewhere or may even seek retribution by filing a malpractice claim. The need to satisfy patients is also fueled by the financial and other rewards given by managed care companies and health systems to those physicians and medical groups that score well on patient satisfaction surveys. Those incentives and the publication, by practice, of regional and national patient satisfaction survey results provide data that are difficult to dismiss or dispute.

"One size fits all" satisfaction strategies cannot work for every patient because preferences are created and altered by individual experiences and influences. What does work is identifying and managing patient expectations and knowing how to respond to unmet expectations. This book focuses on these critical elements of a patient satisfaction effort.

Who Should Read This Book

The purpose of *Managing Patient Expectations* is to help physicians, clinicians, and those who work with them in outpatient settings to understand and respond to the needs and preferences that patients bring to the physician-patient relationship.

This book will be of interest to individuals who hold leadership positions in health care systems. To be successful, their organizations need delivery networks that meet patient expectations for service and clinical excellence. The financial losses associated with patients with unmet expectations who choose to seek care elsewhere are significant. Organizations seeking national quality awards must document their processes and the results of identifying, managing, and reconciling differing patient expectations.

Managing patient expectations is critically important for individuals with case management responsibilities in organizations assuming risk. Case managers have the challenging role of educating both patients and physicians about available resources. Patient expectations have been a barrier to changing physician behavior. Nearly every physician has given a prescription, extended a hospital stay, or ordered a test because the patient expected it—and it was easier to abide by the patient's wishes than to take the time to manage the patient's expectations. This book provides low-cost, realistic strategies that can be quickly implemented in the medical setting.

Managing Patient Expectations is also written for risk managers who know that satisfied patients do not sue and that strong physician-patient relationships prevent malpractice claims.

Professionals interested in patient outcomes will benefit from reading this book. Managing patient expectations is a useful strategy in achieving better outcomes. When patients are asked to assess their level of function or their ability to carry on activities of daily living, expectations will play a critical role in their assessment.

Physician assistants, nurse practitioners, psychologists, therapists, and other clinicians who work in private practice and other outpatient settings and want to create positive and realistic patient expectations will also be interested in this book.

Overview of the Contents

The first step in managing patient expectations is to understand how they are created. The chapters in Part One consider the expectations that arise from the patient's experiences, from word of mouth, from media and advertising exposure, and from first impressions.

The second step in managing expectations is to identify them. Part Two discusses the listening skills you can use to determine expectations and the benefits of obtaining patient feedback.

In medicine, as in every other profession and industry, it is not possible to satisfy every patient's every preference. Part Three focuses on key strategies to manage patient expectations.

Technical and diagnostic skills are important, but patients do not assess them as quickly as they do the quality of the interactions between the physician and staff and the patient and family. Those interactions are moments of truth, and they need to be exemplary in conveying interest, understanding, empathy, and compassion. Chapter Eight describes this concept of moments of truth.

The vital role that every staff member plays in managing patient expectations is the focus of Chapter Nine. Medical visits are, after all, meetings of people. Medicine is a relationship business, made or broken by the people in it. Chapter Ten addresses the value of informed consent in helping patients have realistic expectations. Patient education is addressed in Chapter Eleven. Chapter Twelve reviews techniques used by successful companies to identify and respond to customer expectations.

Part Four examines typical situations in which patient expectations are unmet. Some patients have unrealistic expectations that cannot be met. They do not want to be as good as new; they want to be better than new. They expect their physicians to be available twenty-four hours a day, seven days a week. They do not expect to pay a bill, because their insurance covers everything. When expectations are not met, a patient may choose to complain or seek care elsewhere. Chapter Thirteen identifies the principles of effective complaint handling.

Chapter Fourteen considers issues of patient follow-through with the agreed-upon treatment plan. Although level of follow-through is often linked with outcome, not all patients recover from their illnesses. Even when the highest quality of care has been provided, outcomes may be less than the patient and family expected. When a mistake has occurred, physicians and other members of the organization may react emotionally and make a difficult situation worse. Chapter Fifteen discusses techniques for handling the adverse outcome. Chapter Sixteen focuses on communication with patients who have left the practice.

We place great value on relationships in which our unique needs are identified and respected. Part Five focuses on how physicians can respect patients' individual preferences and build relationships with patients that are rewarding for physician and patient both.

Acknowledgments

Many friends and colleagues have offered advice or encouragement at various points in the process of writing this book. I would like to thank the following people:

Joan and Paul Keane, my parents, and Barbara Cochran, Athena DuFresne, and Paul R. Keane, my siblings, for their love and support.

Angela Cesa, for being a wise and wonderful friend.

Sister Daniel Marie McCabe, Maria R. Morris, and Claude E. Padgett for their willingness to share the knowledge they have gained in their distinguished careers. It has been my great privilege to work for them.

Lisa Anthony, John V. Campano, Beatrice C. Holt, Martha Dale, Martin Fink, Frank J. Hannon, Susan Hostage, Beverly Jacobson, Thomas Lynch, Joseph Mailloux, William McDonough, John Meehan, Phyllis Russell, Arthur Sampson, Louis Schenkel, and Marcie Shepard for their early support and continuing interest in my efforts to promote the value of creating positive relationships in the medical setting.

Alvin L. Morris for proving to me once and for all what I have always suspected: the most talented people are also the most gracious.

Jonathan Goldweitz, my physician, for being there whenever my family and I have needed him for the past eighteen years. He has taught us a great deal about the dignity of the physician-patient relationship.

Adrienne Chieng, Liz Kramer, and Andy Pasternak for their editorial support, which has been both helpful and reassuring.

Marianne Bo, Richard Commaille, Judith DiPasquale, Mary Judge, Gail Kennerknecht, Sister Therese Landry, Lucille Lieberman, Sandra Malloy, Frank McKernan, and Merill Ann Weinstein, with whom I have had the good fortune of working during my career, for the examples they have set and the expertise they have shared, and for their encouragement.

Ann Callahan for her friendship and generosity. Without her helpful input and review throughout the development of the manuscript, *Managing Patient Expectations* might never have been completed.

June 1998   Susan Keane Baker
                                    New Canaan, Connecticut

For
George, Jane, and Thomas Baker
You are everything a family should be

The Author

. . . .

Susan Keane Baker speaks and writes about patient satisfaction and risk management issues. Her seminars have been presented to more than twenty-five thousand health care professionals. She is a frequent speaker for hospitals, insurance companies, group practices, professional societies, and managed care organizations.

Baker works with Metropolitan Life's ten-million-member PPO, where she is responsible for quality improvement and patient satisfaction systems. From 1977 to 1995, she held vice president and senior vice president positions at hospitals in Connecticut and New York.

Baker is a fellow of the American College of Healthcare Executives and a fellow of the American Society for Healthcare Risk Management. She is on the faculty for the Healthcare Assembly's Physician Practice Management Certificate Program. She teaches graduate seminars in practice management for Fairfield University and Quinnipiac College. She serves as the practice management consultant for *Advance for Nurse Practitioners* and *Advance for Physician Assistants*. Her columns appear regularly in those journals and in *American Medical News*.

A cum laude graduate of the College of the Holy Cross, she received her master's degree in health services administration from the State University of New York, Stony Brook. Baker works in New Canaan, Connecticut, and can be reached at 203-966-4880.

Managing Patient
Expectations

. . . .

· ·

Introduction

*A life isn't significant except for its impact on
other lives.*

Jackie Robinson

It's Monday morning. Last night, you read the latest research study on patient satisfaction. According to the authors, patients want evening appointments, sufficient time with their doctor, and no payment at the time of service. Your assistant tells you that Mrs. Cole is waiting. Ah, Mrs. Cole. Your patient who wants only 9:00 A.M. appointments, begins to fidget if the visit goes on longer than fifteen minutes, and always wants to "settle up the account" before she leaves the office.

Research studies are often valuable sources of information, and you will find references to dozens of them in this book. Research helps you identify changes in preferences and expectations of patients like those you care for in your practice. However, it is not enough to consider the average expectations of a group of patients. To build loyal patient relationships, you must meet or manage the specific expectations of each patient. Patient satisfaction research can offer only minimal insight into the individuality of any given patient. No research study will pinpoint the expectations of a specific patient in your practice. Expectations are created and altered by a person's experiences and influences, including current somatic symptoms; perceived vulnerability to illness; past experiences; and knowledge acquired from physicians, friends, family, or the media (Kravitz and others, 1996). The goal of this book is to provide you with strategies to identify and respond to each patient's expectations.

Expectations Defined

Expectations arise continually throughout a person's life, developing from beliefs and values based on impressions and experiences. Unique to an individual, they determine one's perceptions of what is to come (Oscar, 1996). Expectations "primarily reflect an expectancy, a perception that the occurrence of a given event is likely. Thus patient expectations are anticipations that given events are likely to occur during, or as a result of, medical care" (Uhlmann, Inui, and Carter, 1984, p. 681). Expectations are not the same as preferences. For example, patients may expect to feel pain after surgery, but that does not mean that they want or prefer pain. We will be looking at both positive and negative expectations in this book.

Expectations can affect a patient's decision to seek care. In one study, patients were asked about their expectations about symptoms associated with an impending myocardial infarction. Of the patients studied, 74 percent had symptoms that were different from what they expected, and these patients waited significantly longer to obtain treatment (Johnson and King, 1995). Further understanding of patients' expectations could improve the clinical process of care, health care delivery systems, and health services research (Kravitz and others, 1996).

Expectations and Satisfaction

Our satisfaction with most encounters, medical or otherwise, often depends on whether or not our expectations are met. The purpose of managing expectations is to have as little discrepancy as possible between patients' expectations and their actual experience. Maintaining a balance of consistency and flexibility allows you to accomplish this.

Successful companies deliver products that are designed and delivered to meet customer expectations. The quality of what they provide has two dimensions: product quality and service quality. Richard C. Whiteley (1991), author of *The Customer Driven Company*, defines product as "what you get" and service as "how you get it." We can say that *quality* means meeting both your expectations for technical competence and your patient's expectations as defined in the context of his or her own experience.

Understanding how expectations are created, responding to those expectations, and influencing expectations are important factors in developing mutually beneficial relationships with your patients. Studies have found that meeting patient expectations correlates positively with high satisfaction (Williams, Weinman, Dale, and Newman, 1995). Although that sounds like a report from the department of the obvious, most physicians will admit that they do not take time to ask patients if their expectations for care are being met. Instead, many physicians develop systems and communication styles that they think are effective, then wait for occasional feedback that supports their decisions. For years, physicians held tight to the notion that they knew best. Patient suggestions about their medical care were often dismissed with the pilot analogy: "Patients should no more tell a doctor how to practice medicine than airline passengers should tell a pilot how to fly a plane." Today, increasingly knowledgeable patients fully expect that you will discuss their needs and preferences with them.

Patients and Customers

You will find references to customers in this book. The term *customer* offends some physicians, especially those who wish that the traditional physician-patient relationship could be restored. When the word customer is used in this book, it refers to people in non-medical situations. (And while on the subject of language: although the use of "he or she" isn't cumbersome in a brief article, it does become tedious in a book of this length. Therefore, except for specific examples, I will use "he" for patients and "she" for physicians in this text.)

Consistency and Flexibility

The successful practice achieves the balance of consistency and flexibility that provides patients with the security of predictability and the comfort of knowing that they are cared for as individuals, not as symptoms or disease categories. One way to maintain this balance is to make your service as consistent as possible while at the same time customizing the interactions you have with patients. Flexibility is important to patients, particularly those who feel alienated in impersonal relationships with large organizations, such as insurance companies and huge systems. Chapter Eighteen describes a consistency-flexibility model.

None of the ideas in this book requires a team of consultants to implement. Many of the strategies are widely known. However, common knowledge is not common practice. Choosing ten or twenty of the strategies in this book and working with your staff to implement them on a consistent basis will provide your practice with a distinct competitive advantage.

Part I

Creating Expectations

Prior Experiences

*Nothing ever becomes real till it is experienced. Even
a proverb is no Proverb to you till your Life has
illustrated it.*

John Keats

Asking your patients about their prior medical experiences provides them with a nonthreatening way to tell you what they prefer in a physician-patient relationship. In interviews with patients who reported that their expectations for care in an office practice were not met (Kravitz and others, 1996), 42 percent reported that their unmet expectations were shaped by past experiences with similar symptoms or illnesses or by experiences acquired while caring for others. Their personal experiences influenced their expectations for both diagnosis and therapy.

Memories of prior experiences guide patients as they make decisions and consider treatment alternatives. Almost everyone has had some personal experience with the health care system, and the conviction of a prior experience is fierce. If it happened to your patient, he knows it for a fact. In 1997, the State of New Jersey passed legislation requiring insurers to pay for a second day in the hospital for vaginal deliveries and four days for a cesarean section delivery. In considering the issue, Governor Christine Todd Whitman was probably advised that some studies have shown that readmission and complication rates are not higher for women and infants discharged earlier from the hospital. However, her own prior experiences were a factor in her decision to sign the legislation into law. She was quoted as saying, "I've had two children and I know 24 hours is not enough" (Preston, 1997, p. B1).

People who romanticize former times and experiences may seek to duplicate a relationship they remember fondly. Some of your patients want a relationship like one they have had before—even if it was paternalistic. Or they may prefer a certain communication style. A patient might say, "I really liked it when my last physician called me even when my test results were normal."

A patient who has been cared for at a Spence Center for Women's Health in Massachusetts has become accustomed to receiving a terry cloth robe instead of a paper johnnie and has been able to use the telephone provided in the examination room to make local calls while waiting there. She has been cared for in an environment designed to make her feel not just comfortable but pampered. Visiting your practice, this former Spence Center patient probably doesn't expect to receive complimentary bottled water and roasted soybeans. She can obtain those items on her own. However, clinical amenities, if she has developed an expectation of them, will contribute to her satisfaction with your practice. A thirty-seven-year-old patient was impressed when her Spence physician took time to sketch out a diagram of her breasts, illustrating the location of her normal cysts. That was the remarkable moment in her care. Talking for a moment about her experiences would, in all probability, elicit that story. A new physician could then decide to brush up on *her* drawing skills or explain to the patient why she considers such illustrations problematic.

Learning about your patient's experiences with symptoms and illnesses can help you understand what symptoms and illness mean to him. Was the amount of pain most significant to him? Was how soon he could return to work a critical factor in his decision making? In sharing his experiences, or those of significant people in his life, he will frame for you his perceived ability to function in the future. Memories of prior experiences may be inaccurate, or advances may have changed some aspects of what a condition or procedure was like in the past. If the patient has come to see you because of a specific symptom or suspicion of illness, he may have formed some expectations from reading about that condition or speaking with family members or colleagues. Listening to your patient will give you an opportunity to correct any misconceptions he may have.

Prior experiences can have an impact on compliance and outcomes. After unsuccessful treatments, a patient's expectations about outcome may be lower. This could be one reason why repeated back surgeries often lead to progressively poorer results (Benson and Friedman, 1996).

Patients who have elected to visit a number of different doctors for the same complaint may have unrealistic expectations that you will need to address. Regardless of why patients receive care from multiple physicians or organizations, they find it relatively easy to compare physicians and practices. As Samuel Butler said, "The public do not know enough to be experts, yet know enough to decide between them." A patient may perceive two practices as being different as night and day. One patient said of her experience with different practices:

> At the first practice, no one said hello to me or even noticed that I was there. I sat alone like someone waiting for a bus, not someone waiting for an intimate exam. They made me feel as if everything they had to do was more important than me.
>
> At the other practice, the woman who answers the phone is very nice. She doesn't rush you. The doctor is nice too. He warmed the instrument before using it, which wasn't a big deal for me, but I liked his thoughtfulness in thinking of it. They really care about you there.

Note that the quality of the greeting this patient received created an impression that was later confirmed in her mind by her subsequent experiences.

Your patient probably has multiple, and sometimes conflicting, expectations. He may not have prioritized them, and it is a good idea for you to help him do so. For example, you might ask, "What's more important to you, seeing the same doctor every time you visit or obtaining the first available appointment with any of the doctors?"

Prior Experiences with Your Organization

It is important to know if a patient has had prior experiences in your practice or in your system. If you have ever had a problem with an organization and discussed it with a company representative, you might have heard yourself say, "I've been a loyal customer here for eight years, and . . ." Patients know how long they have been in your care, either by date or by a significant event in their life, such as moving to your town, becoming pregnant, suspecting an illness, or changing jobs. Establish a system that tells you how long a patient has been receiving care from you. It need not be as elaborate as the American Express policy of imprinting "Member since 1982" on credit cards. You can color-code your file folders or include a first visit date on the registration page of your patient records.

On occasion, you or your staff may not recognize a patient. Perhaps it has been some time since the last visit, or the patient's name has changed, or the patient is simply unfamiliar for some reason. Instead of asking, "Are you a new patient?" ask, "When was your last visit?" A new patient won't be offended by the question, and you'll avoid offending an established patient. Reviewing the schedule and your patient's prior records before your meeting helps prevent this situation. When you cannot greet your patient by name, listen carefully for the patient to give you his name, and then use it warmly.

Very Important Patients

Some patients will have higher service expectations because of their position in society, particularly if they hold an important role in their health care system. They may expect that their need for care should come before that of other patients. Although you want to provide the same quality of care to all patients, you may choose to offer special accommodations to high-profile patients. One hospital was more than happy to free up adjoining patient rooms for patients' business meetings, arrange for meal delivery from favorite restaurants, and provide special toiletries and fresh flowers. Practices that care for high-profile patients may have private entrances, private office hours, transportation, and a commitment to being on time for appointments. One group asked the VIP's assistant about his favorite music and arranged to have that CD playing when the patient arrived for visits. Discussing your prior experiences in caring for high-profile patients with the patient may help him decide what, if any, special arrangements he prefers. Be sure to alert key team members about any special accommodations you agree to make.

It can be disconcerting for other patients to watch preferential treatment being provided to a high-profile patient, so be as inconspicuous as you can when doing so. Team members may need coaching about why preferential treatment is being given and the need to be discreet about it. Without this coaching, employees may not understand your rationale and speak disparagingly about the patient, you, or the special accommodations. An Alabama hospital had to quickly cancel a special emergency department program offered to its trustees and local elected officials when employees became vocal in their opposition to the preferential treatment plan ("Alabama Hospital's ER Access Program . . . ," 1996). Conversely, staff may gravitate to a celebrity patient, so be conscientious about seeing that appropriate care is provided to other patients on a timely basis.

High-profile patients may request special assurances about the confidentiality of medical information and records. This is a great opportunity for you to evaluate your system for divulging patient information. Good Samaritan Hospital in Los Angeles forbids staff members to speak with the press for any reason. Ann Callahan, former director of marketing and public affairs for Manhattan Eye, Ear, and Throat Hospital, used this response to inquiries about high-profile or celebrity patients: "It is our strict policy not to discuss anything about any of our patients. I'm sure you expect the same courtesy from your physician." Placing emphasis on the word *any* sent a strong and reassuring message to existing and potential patients.

Alternative Therapies

Alternative medicine is gaining widespread acceptance in many communities. An article in *Hospitals and Health Networks* reported that a public clinic for natural medicine was formed in Seattle after a management consultant considering the concept learned that eleven of the thirteen city council members were already receiving some form of natural medicine ("Seattle Goes au Naturel," 1996).

Patients receiving alternative therapy may be reluctant to share that information for fear that you will consider them ignorant or too far from the mainstream. It is important to be nonjudgmental about alternative therapies so that patients feel comfortable about discussing them with you. You do not want to be like the physician who listened to her patient discuss his visits with a faith healer, a palm reader, and a guru. "And," asked the physician, "what foolish advice did they give you?" The patient answered, "They all told me to see you."

Physicians should ask about a patient's use of alternative therapies. Researchers in one study (Eisenberg, 1997) found that 83 percent of patients who were using unconventional therapy for serious medical conditions were obtaining care for the same condition from a medical doctor. But 72 percent of respondents failed to inform their physician that they were doing so. Recognizing this phenomenon, many physicians are now more open to understanding the practices of other caregivers. Respecting, or at least not dismissing, alternative forms of healing can help the physician and patient work together so that the patient has a reasonable plan of treatment. Patients are more likely to follow through with your treatment plan if it accommodates their alternative therapy.

The media have focused on patient satisfaction with alternative medicine, rather than its clinical outcomes. The popularity of alternative medicine despite the lack of scientific proof about its effectiveness speaks to the idea that if patients believe in the process they will be satisfied with the outcome. Physicians should encourage patients who are interested in alternative therapies to choose licensed providers, document their symptoms, and return to the physician for follow-up care (Eisenberg, 1997). Showing respect for an alternative healer may influence not only your patient but his healer as well.

Beliefs

Beliefs are often the determining factor in patient follow-through and outcomes. Since the first studies of placebos, physicians have recognized the significant role of patient beliefs in the physician-patient relationship. A physical placebo is not always necessary to evoke a placebo effect. "Three components are necessary: (a) positive beliefs and expectations on the part of the patient; (b) positive beliefs and expectations on the part of the physician or health care professional; and (c) a good relationship between both parties" (Benson and Friedman, 1996, p. 193). One example of a nonphysical placebo is "that moment when providers and patients agree on expectations. . . . Providers are likely to focus on delivering the expected outcomes and patients are preprogrammed to receive them. Patients experience the outcomes they expect, because they expect them" (MacStravic, 1989, p. 53).

Understanding religious beliefs can be important in treatment planning, but appreciating the role of religious beliefs can be difficult for clinicians who are not religious themselves. Dale A. Matthews of Georgetown University reviewed 212 studies on the influence of religious belief on health ("Studies Suggest Religious Activities Can Improve Health," 1996). Three-quarters of the studies showed a positive effect of religion on health, whereas only 7 percent concluded that religion had had a negative impact on health. Churches often provide strong support networks. Some patients have healthier lifestyles because they abide by religious prohibitions against the use of alcohol and tobacco. Although religious beliefs can provide clues about motivation, you should not make assumptions based on religious affiliations alone. For example, individuals may elect to receive blood products or to use birth control, despite their religious beliefs.

• • • • • • •

Learning about your patient's life experiences is an important strategy in identifying the expectations against which you will be evaluated.

Questions you can use to determine expectations created by patients' prior experiences include the following:

- Would you tell me about experiences you have had as a patient that were pleasing for you?

- What's the most important quality you are looking for in a physician?

- What's the second most important quality you are looking for in a physician?

- How have physicians been helpful to you?

- Why have you decided to choose a new physician?

- Have you ever had an experience like this before?

Second in importance to the conviction of a patient's own experiences is what he has learned from credible people in his life. The expectations created by word of mouth are discussed in the next chapter.

3

Word of Mouth

*What people say behind your back is your standing in
the community.*

Edgar Watson Howe

A few years ago, Denise Cavanaugh, a consultant with Cavanaugh, Hagan & Pierson in Washington, D.C., told the story
of two men who were the youngest ever graduates of the academy
at West Point to be installed as army generals. A reporter from
Time interviewed them and asked, "What do you think of this
coincidence that the two of you would be made the youngest generals during the same year?" It wasn't a coincidence, the men responded. At graduation from the academy, the two agreed that
wherever they went during their careers, they would tell people of
the other's accomplishments. The man stationed in Germany often
spoke well of the man in Washington and vice versa. This happened
again and again as they moved from post to post, from rank to rank
(Denise Cavanaugh, personal communication with the author,
1992).

You hope that people speak well of the care and service your
practice provides. When they do, patients choose you because they
want you—because what they have heard about your practice is all
they need to know to believe that you are the right physician for

them. You are fortunate when patients select you on the basis of word of mouth, because they have a sense of what to expect. Individuals who are referred are more likely to be satisfied, because they tend to be like the person who referred them. Referred people stay longer than those who respond to advertising, sales pitches, or price promotions (Reichheld, 1996).

The more information patients have about you, the more likely they are to be satisfied with their experience. Joseph Wassersug, a retired internist living in Boca Raton, Florida, refers to this concept as the "recognition factor." When a new patient says, "I know you; you're the doctor who . . . ," the patient is more receptive to you. If they have heard of you, they think you're good (Joseph Wassersug, letter to the author, 1998). A Kaiser Family Foundation and Agency for Healthcare Policy and Research study (1996) found that three out of four respondents would prefer a surgeon they were acquainted with to an unfamiliar one, even if the unfamiliar physician had a higher rating of some kind. Wassersug advises working with your hospital marketing department; writing a book, article, or letter to the editor; and being involved with the community as strategies to increase community awareness about you and your practice.

What do your patients say about you? Patients do not recommend your practice by saying, "Go to Dr. Petrie's office, they always answer the phone," or, "Maura Smith is a great nurse practitioner; she always puts a bandage on your arm after drawing blood." Patients comment on what impresses them, such as a presurgical or postvisit telephone call, or that you really take time to listen.

Every successful organization has leadership that realizes it cannot be everything to everyone. Decide what you want to be known for. Writing down the answers to the following questions can help you determine this:

- What is it about your organization that makes it different?

- Who should choose your practice rather than others in your area?

- What do you have to offer that your competitors do not have?

- What is special about the way you conduct business?

- What would you like people to know about you that they do not know now?

- What is it about your practice that offers greater advantages, benefits, or results for your patients?

Rarely can anyone respond to these questions quickly. If you want your patients, employees, and referral sources to be able to answer these questions, you have to supply them with information. List the services that your practice provides, and identify the exceptional characteristics of each. For whom are those services best suited? When you choose the components of service or value that you want to emphasize, you can raise patient expectations in that particular area.

You can shape patient expectations by stressing the benefit of what differentiates your practice. If you always find room in the schedule for patients in pain, let people know. If you excel at convenience, you'll attract patients who value convenience. If you respond quickly to patients, you'll attract patients who value speed and responsiveness. One physician was committed to seeing her patients on schedule. Patients were advised that if they arrived more than fifteen minutes after their appointment time, they would be offered another appointment or the option of waiting until there was a lull in the schedule. If expert advice is your strength, you can attract patients who want more detailed information. What do your preferred patients value? What can you do to offer that value in a manner superior to others who provide the same services you do? What examples can you use to illustrate your niche to patients, staff, and others who refer patients to you?

Negative Impressions

Is there anything worse than a patient who says, "I go to Dr. Jones, but I wouldn't recommend him." What impression do you want people to take away as a result of your life's work? That you would have been happier if you had gone to business school? Be honest. Are you spending more time complaining about managed care than you are talking about the strengths of your practice? Many patients are tired of hearing a diatribe of complaints about something over which they have no control.

Sometimes, it is best *not* to say what is on your mind. You tend to talk about what you are thinking about, but sometimes talking about what is on your mind gives the patient the wrong impression. There's an old story about a physician sitting with his patient the night before surgery. To ease her fears, he begins telling her about the costs of his daughter's wedding and his son's college tuition. As he is leaving, he asks, "Do you have any questions?" "Just one," the patient replies, "Am I paying for the college or the wedding?"

What Do Your Staff Members Tell Others About You?

"My doctor's very good; his secretary said so," a woman replied when asked about her physician. The most effective word of mouth is what your staff have to say about your practice. After all, staff members know the inside story. Is each member of your team an advocate for your practice all the time or just when you are around? Do staff members understand how important they are in creating positive impressions about the practice?

You have less to fear from your competitors than from indifference or negativity on the part of members of your own practice. Listen and respond to employee shop talk. Observe what kinds of comments are being made. Researchers from the University of Pennsylvania and the University of Pittsburgh rode in hospital elevators to observe the discussions being held there (Ubel and others, 1995). In 14 percent of the elevator trips, researchers heard inappropriate comments, and half of those involved breaches of patient confidentiality. Physicians were observed talking about making large amounts of money; administrators discussed a death that was the hospital's mistake; nurses talked about whether a colleague was too ill to assist in a procedure.

> **You have less to fear from your competitors than from indifference or negativity on the part of members of your own practice.**

Unprofessional Comments

Criticizing other people reaches epidemic proportions in some organizations. In addition to creating a discouraging atmosphere, it is very upsetting to patients who overhear comments, or worse, who are the audience for critical remarks about others. A patient spoke of seeing a physician who was part of a small group practice. The physician was being extremely critical of the senior physician. She did not criticize his clinical skills but the way he treated her and women in general. Did this have anything to do with the purpose of the patient's visit? No, and it made the patient feel uncomfortable enough to look for a new physician.

These examples remind me of my mother's advice: "Don't bother people with your problems, because 90 percent of them don't care and the other 10 percent are glad you have them."

Staff Comments

What do your staff members tell patients about you? In one practice, the physician takes every Tuesday off in order to be with his young children. Staff members take pride in working for this man, and their sentiments are shared by his patients, who don't expect to reach him on Tuesdays. Another physician, Wayne Peters, was honored by 350 residents of Middlebury, Vermont. His office manager shared her favorite story about him with a reporter from the *New York Times* ("Town Thanks Its Doctor . . . ," 1996). A woman delivered a baby prematurely on a hiking trail in the mountains. Peters hiked up the mountain with an incubator, put the baby in it, and hiked back down. "He'd go anywhere to see a patient," the office manager said. Of course, the stories don't have to be just about you. Make it a point to share positive information about your staff with colleagues, patients, family members, and friends.

Stories help people make connections because people remember stories much more easily than a list of facts. Using customer stories has been a very successful strategy for Patagonia, the sports apparel company. Patagonia found that focusing on how customers feel and behave provides valuable insight for product development and encourages increased customer feedback. What are the stories told about your practice? When you are hosting a holiday, retirement, or other party, listen carefully to the stories that are told and retold. If the majority are about mistakes, incompetence, or conflict, it's time for you to tell a few stories of your own about positive differences staff members have made in the lives of your patients.

It takes some maturity and experience in several different work settings before some employees realize that every organization has faults. If a few younger employees are not referring new patients to you, they probably haven't thought much about it or don't know what to say. However, if the majority of your employees are not recommending new patients, something is wrong. There is most likely a quality issue that you have not faced up to or remedied. Employees want to be proud of their organization, and if they have concerns, they will be reluctant to invite their friends and associates to become patients.

Referral Sources

Every person who comes to you on the basis of a referral rather than having selected you from the yellow pages or a health plan directory is likely to be a better-informed patient. That person knows something about you and has formed some expectations. Most physician referral services are eager to make appropriate referrals to your practice. When you develop a relationship with its staff members, a referral service can be like having a paid advertising agency for your practice. The referral service staff will spend the time necessary to identify patient preferences and help your new patient know what to expect.

Do not assume that because you have hospital privileges or belong to the medical society that you are registered with the organization's referral service. The service may have sent you a letter of invitation that you overlooked or did not receive. Make an appointment to meet with the referral staff. Understand the process of how referrals are made. Ask about the most frequently received requests made by callers to the service.

Preparing Your Profile

Referral services maintain standard profiles to answer the questions asked most frequently by patients. You can expect to provide information about your specialty, education, board certification, office location(s), office hours, accepted insurance plans, access for patients with disabilities, and languages you speak fluently. You might also be asked (or you might want) to provide information on whether you make house calls, whether you accept patients who request not to receive blood or blood products, and other items of interest.

Prepare responses that accurately reflect what patients will experience. Remember to consider the talents of your staff when completing the profile. The questionnaire may ask about languages in which you are fluent. Your response could be, "The physician is fluent in English, and the full-time registered nurse is fluent in English and Spanish." When completing your profile, add information that might be helpful or make you more memorable. When the referral staff are speaking with a prospective patient, it is possible that they will use your own words, so position your information in the most favorable way possible. For example, when identifying your location you might simply list your address. Or you could list your address and enhance it by adding, "Free parking next to building."

After you complete the referral profile, sit down with the referral service coordinator to review it. He or she may mention information that you can add to your profile. Mary Judge, supervisor of physician relations at the Stamford Hospital, Stamford, Connecticut, says that the request she receives most frequently is for "a doctor who listens." She has been asked to recommend physicians who understand the problems of alcoholism, physicians who have a special interest in adolescents, chronic fatigue syndrome, cholesterol, Lyme disease, obesity, massage therapy, and vitamins. She has also received requests for offices that are convenient to public transportation and for practices that do not use voice mail (Mary Judge, telephone interview with author, 1997).

Building Relationships with Referral Staff

Keep in mind that when you meet with the referral staff, they may have their own agenda. They may want to tell you about changes or new services at their organization. Be receptive. You want to cultivate a mutually beneficial relationship. You can also use the time to talk with the referral coordinator about the kinds of patients you would most like to attract.

Always thank the person who refers a patient to your practice, whether or not the patient actually visits you. And be sure to acknowledge the value of the service to the manager of the program.

If your hospital or health system has a physician referral program, invite referral staff to spend time in your organization. If you participate with a referral service located in another area of the country, it will take a little more initiative to establish a relationship with the staff there. The representative who meets with you in your office is probably not the same person who will be answering calls from prospective patients. Send photographs of you, your staff, your building, your community. Include the referral staff on your mailing list to receive newsletters, holiday cards, and so on. Sending a note of appreciation to referral staff in a remote location is an effective way to build a relationship.

Keeping Your Profile Accurate

Judge also advises that it is important to update your profile on a regular basis. If you offer Saturday office hours and then discontinue them, you will disappoint patients who select you because of their preference to be seen on that day. Even if the patient decides to continue with you, he will have a nagging suspicion that the rest of your profile may be flawed as well. Whenever you make or anticipate changes, take the time to notify your referral service. A telephone call to alert the referral staff of something as basic as a change of area code can give the impression of a well-run practice. Following up with a note increases the likelihood that the change will be recorded according to your wishes.

Double-check your profile. If you participate with managed care companies that provide information on complication rates or patient satisfaction survey results, be sure that the information is current and accurate. Confirm your participation in managed care plans with both the customer service and medical management divisions of the company.

A health plan member was given the names of several centers when her child needed physical therapy. She took time off from her job to visit each organization before selecting one. Having made her choice, she asked the child's physician to obtain approval. The response from the managed care company's medical management department was that she could not use any of the physical therapy centers that had been identified by the company's customer service department. In fact, the only physical therapy service she could use was one that customer service didn't even have on its list. Her time and energy wasted, she felt angry when she brought her child to the center for treatment.

Managed care companies often encourage patients to schedule get-acquainted visits to see the practice and meet the physicians. Yes, these meetings take time, and no, you usually don't get paid for it. But it provides you with a valuable opportunity to see if a visitor is someone you would like to have as a patient. If a health plan sponsors tours of network provider sites for its staff members, participate. Be more than a listing in a directory whenever you can.

Informal Referral Sources

Each community has informal referral sources, such as local clergy, real estate agents, newcomers groups, lawyers, community leaders, fire and police officers, and people who supply medical products or services. These individuals often have larger spheres of influence than other people. In one community, the newcomers group representative routinely welcomed new homeowners with the following advice: "Look up the telephone number for a private ambulance and keep it by your phone because the town ambulance will only take you to XYZ Hospital, and you do not, under any circumstances, want to go to their emergency department."

Discover what your local chamber of commerce has to offer. Becoming involved in chamber activities should result in patient referrals. But even if you never attract one new patient this way, what you will learn about customer service and demographic trends will make the investment of your time worthwhile.

Almost anyone working in a health care setting is viewed as a credible source of inside information. A man who needed surgery asked everyone even remotely involved in medicine to name three excellent surgeons. After surveying seven or eight people, he took the most frequently mentioned name and felt confident about choosing that surgeon. Listen for the comments of patients about whether they chose you because of, or in spite of, this sort of word of mouth.

Let people know how to refer a prospective patient to your practice. Referral cards should include telephone numbers, directions or maps, and office hours. Some practices volunteer to contact patients who have been referred but have not followed through to make an appointment.

Establish relationships with staff members of physicians who refer patients to you. Acknowledge them by name when you call, and thank them for any referrals they make. Some physicians maintain unlisted telephone numbers for referral sources to use so that they can quickly schedule appointments for their patients. Host a meeting or party at your office and invite referring physicians and their staff members. Consider this scenario: a prospective patient says to the receptionist at his primary care office: "I have the names of two specialists. Do you know either of them?" The receptionist responds, "Well, I don't know Dr. Johnson, but Dr. Lowe over on Maple Street is very nice." Which physician is the patient likely to choose?

Patients: Your Sales Team

A patient is most likely to tell other people about you in the first fourteen days after a visit with you (Cafferky, 1994). Communicating with your patient during that time increases the odds that he will tell others about you.

In order to make effective comments about you, patients must have positive experiences in your care. Although positive word of mouth won't guarantee that a prospective patient will choose you, negative word of mouth essentially guarantees that he won't. If a patient has had a negative experience in your care, resolving the issue quickly and fairly is very important. Effective complaint handling is discussed in Chapter Thirteen.

What is remarkable, special, or consistent about your practice that patients might comment on? One physician takes time to personally schedule the next appointment with her patients. She finds that the time she spends with the patient during those scheduling moments is another opportunity to understand her patient's lifestyle and stresses. My internist is very personable; he gives me his undivided attention and always seems to understand how I feel. When I refer someone to him, I usually mention that he comes out to the reception area to greet his patients. To me, this act of courtesy represents all of his fine qualities. My comments are typical. In an article in *American Medical News*, Charles Atkins (1997, p. 29) wrote, "I listen to my patients talk about their doctors, the good ones and the bad ones—patients are seldom ambivalent about their physicians. What comes across are the intangibles, not how skillfully someone prescribes a beta blocker or inserts a catheter during angioplasty, but how much caring and concern the patient perceives in the doctor's demeanor." Many patients do not understand the technical aspects of medicine, but they do understand sensitivity and courtesy.

Extremely thoughtful gestures almost always generate positive word of mouth. A child was slightly injured when her parents were out of town for the afternoon. The baby-sitter didn't know who the child's pediatrician was and decided to call the pediatrician of another family for whom she worked. She was advised to bring the child to the office, but before she did, the child's mother arrived home. The child was taken to her regular pediatrician. That evening, the mother was amazed to receive a telephone call from the first pediatrician, calling to make sure that the child had received medical attention and was feeling better. The mother is a successful real estate agent in the community, meeting dozens of new families each year. When people ask her to recommend a pediatrician, she speaks glowingly about this physician whom she has never even met.

My Aunt Mary died recently after being homebound for several years and in a nursing home for the last few weeks of her life. While waiting for the undertaker to arrive, Uncle Henry realized that he had an appointment scheduled with his physician on the same day as the funeral. When he called to change his appointment, the receptionist asked him why he wanted to postpone the appointment. "Well, my wife Mary died a few hours ago, and the funeral will be that day," he responded. The receptionist offered sympathy and rescheduled the appointment. Half an hour later, Uncle Henry's physician, who was not Aunt Mary's physician, called him to express his condolences. That story was told and retold at the funeral services. A surprising number of people hearing the story said, "You know, I'm looking for a doctor. Is he taking new patients?"

Learning from Your Best Patients

How can you influence patients to come back again and again? To tell stories about the care they receive from you? To try new services you offer? William H. Davidow and Bro Uttal, coauthors of *Total Customer Service* (1989), recommend that you ask your *best* customers to describe exactly what kind of service they expect. Then ask the customers if they recommend your organization to others. If they do not, find out why. If they do, find out why. One physician learned that some of his patients were not referring others to him because he didn't have a female physician in the group. He decided to promote the availability and talents of the female nurse practitioner in his office.

Acknowledging Referrals

Do patients know that referrals are appreciated? Some practices have a line on their registration form that reads, "Who may we thank for referring you?" This is preferable to a line that reads, "Referred by," because it lets the patient know that you will acknowledge the referral. Acknowledging referrals is a proven strategy for increasing future referrals, but be sure that you have the patient's permission. A neighbor asked me to suggest a plastic surgeon for a friend of hers who wanted a breast augmentation. I received a note from the surgeon thanking me for referring my neighbor, who hadn't shared with me that she was considering the procedure for herself.

How should you thank patients who refer others to your practice? The degree of appreciation depends on your own style. Some physicians clip a note to the referring patient's chart so that they can mention it when they next see the patient. Others send a handwritten note, which is preferable to a computer-generated form letter.

One physician sends, for every five referrals, a beautiful and distinctive coffee mug filled with flowers. The flowers are delivered to the person at work, just before noon, thus guaranteeing that the physician will be a topic of conversation at lunch. The coffee mug has no advertising on it, except on the bottom of the mug, which reads, "Thank you from Dr. Jones, 555-6677." The physician knows that the message is seen whenever the coffee mug is washed or in the dishwasher. He is convinced that people are actively scouting for referrals in order to increase the size of their coffee mug collections.

Giving gifts to patients for referrals can be a delicate matter, because gifts can be misinterpreted. Whereas one patient enjoys receiving a coffee mug or a coupon for a complimentary video rental, another feels offended. Your knowledge of your patient should be your guide. Does your patient have a favorite charity? A contribution in your patient's name would certainly be a memorable gesture of appreciation.

Tracking Referrals

Your staff should compile the number and sources of referrals on a monthly basis and compare them both on a year-to-date basis and with the same month of the prior year. Declining referral patterns should serve as a warning that shifts are occurring that will significantly affect your practice.

• • • • • •

People want to know what their credible friends and associates think about your practice before they commit their time and health to you. When you have strong word of mouth in your favor, you have earned the most valuable kind of advertising. You can't buy it, but if you have earned it, you can take it to the bank.

Advertising, Media, and Managed Care

Half the work done in the world is to make things
appear what they are not.

E. R. Beadle

Today, advertising, media, and managed care each contribute significantly to the expectations patients have about medical care. Advertisements and marketing efforts have flourished as competition for patients has escalated. The *Wall Street Journal* (Jeffrey, 1996) reported that in 1995, hospital advertising expenditures exceeded $1 billion. Organizations touted their names, staff members, missions, and patient satisfaction scores, all the while creating expectations that were often impossible for those actually providing the care to fulfill.

Advertising

Good advertising creates realistic expectations while helping patients access your organization with minimal difficulty. A good advertisement is one that attracts people's attention and moves them to a decision they feel good about, one they believe will be of personal benefit to them. The best advertising tells patients what the experience will be like, increasing the likelihood that their expectations will be met.

What does your advertising say about you? It should be sending the exact message you want patients to receive, but does it? Coupons and newspaper advertisements promising a discount or a free service "for new patients only" may convey that you are hungry for business when your intent is to say that you welcome new patients. Marketing experts refer to "new patient only" promotions as death wish strategies. Do you really want to attract a patient who is willing to switch physicians because of a coupon?

Do not create advertisements that promise more than you can deliver. The Club Med resort company was the subject of a *Wall Street Journal* article (Stevens, 1997) after unmarried customers began complaining that instead of the singles dating scene promised in ads, they found themselves vacationing with lots of families with small children. The gap between expectations and reality became newsworthy when a woman visited a Club Med resort to meet handsome, single men in their thirties but instead met balding dads, dozens of kids, and a convention of salesmen from a Brazilian washing machine company. Although she admitted that the reservations clerk had mentioned there would be families at the resort, she wasn't advised that the majority of men would have their own schedule of activities and speak only Portuguese.

Advertisements for plastic surgeons often promise perfection. Do all of their patients look like their advertisements' perfect physical specimens? God doesn't promise perfection, but ads often do and create unrealistic expectations in the process.

The advertisement of James J. Reardon, M.D., a New York City plastic surgeon, is an excellent example of how an advertisement can be used to inform or remind patients about what can be rationally expected after a surgical procedure. Instead of promising restored youth or physical perfection, the ad refers to "the art of aging well." Prospective patients learn that after surgery, "you look like yourself, only better—more rested and refreshed." Dr. Reardon's ad includes his photograph, another good technique for helping patients know what to expect.

Because patients frequently mention the importance of being listened to, some organizations are stressing the ability of their staff to do just that. The Advocate Health Care System in Oak Brook, Illinois, ran print ads featuring pictures of ears. Radio advertisements for Women and Infants Hospital in Rhode Island promise that its physicians understand the unspoken message behind what patients actually say to them.

Patients have perceived little difference among health plans and no connection between their needs and the benefits of managed care. Much of the media coverage about managed care has been negative, and managed care companies have responded with ads that promise a highly satisfying experience. Television and radio commercials for managed care organizations promise beautiful, caring moments for patients choosing their company. As managed care organizations continue to raise the bar regarding the level of service patients should expect from health care organizations, some patients may begin to wonder if other practices are providing more. They may remain loyal to you for their care, but the result of their uncertainty may be that they do not refer others to you.

It is unfortunate the managed care company advertisements fail to educate patients about the realities of managed care: in-network versus out-of-network providers, preauthorizations, alternate benefit and nonduplication of benefit provisions. No component of the health care delivery system takes responsibility for managing patient expectations, leaving patients to anticipate an experience like that promoted in the advertising. The backlash against managed care is the result of unmet expectations, particularly regarding access.

Good advertising provides the kind of information that helps new patients feel confident about how to work with your practice. The Knight's Inn hotel chain uses advertising to attract long-distance truckers, a very loyal group, to stay at their hotels. Their advertisements identify every property with the address, telephone number, room rate, and whether a trucker can park his tractor and trailer rigs on the site. Health care advertisements that provide maps, telephone numbers, participating health plans, exact services offered, information about how to make an appointment, and so on help patients make correct choices. The goal of your advertising should be to help patients feel comfortable, knowing that they are doing the right thing.

You must live up to your advertising, because patients expect the experience to match the rhetoric. When United Airlines advertised, "Fly the friendly skies," their flight attendants had to be friendly. If you promise, "Where the extraordinary happens every day," you have to see to it that patients experience something they perceive as extraordinary. Otherwise, patients with unmet expectations will use your own rhetoric to discredit you.

Patient Bill of Rights

A Patient Bill of Rights can be extremely helpful in educating patients about what they can expect. It is important for you to be very familiar with the Patient Bill of Rights issued to your patients by hospitals, managed care companies, and associations. Patients who read them develop expectations. Exhibit 4.1 is an example of an excellent Patient Bill of Rights; it was developed for children and adolescents by BayState Medical Center in Springfield, Massachusetts.

Media

Stories in the media seek to inform and entertain readers. Although the media have greatly expanded their coverage of medicine, time and space constraints limit how thoroughly an issue can be addressed. Media coverage of the latest advances in medicine can create misplaced enthusiasm and unrealistic expectations on the part of patients. Looking to interest readers, reporters will often focus on a medical breakthrough, with only minor mention that widespread availability is years away or that the drug or procedure will benefit only a small number of people.

Exhibit 4.1. Bill of Rights for Children and Teens.

Respect and Personal Dignity

You are important. We want to get to know you.

We will tell you who we are, and we will call you by your name. We will take time to listen to you.

We won't talk about you in your room or outside your door unless you know what is happening.

We Will Honor Your Privacy

Care that supports you and your family.

You and your family are important. We will work together to make you as safe and comfortable as possible.

All families are different. We want to learn about what's important to you and your family.

There will be a place for a member of your family to spend the night with you or near you.

Information You Can Understand

We will explain things to you. We will speak in ways you can understand. You can ask about what is happening to you and why.

Someone who speaks your language will help explain things to you.

Someone from your family can be with you when people are explaining things to you.

Quality Health Care

You will be taken care of by doctors, nurses, and other people who know about children and teenagers.

You have the right to know all of the people who take care of you. You and your family can meet with them to plan what is best for you.

We will work together with you and your family to make your stay as short and as comfortable as possible.

Emotional Support

When you are in our facility, you might feel scared, mad, lonely, or sad. You can let people know how you feel. It is okay to cry or complain.

You can have your family with you as much as possible. When this is not possible, the other people caring for you will explain why.

We can help you meet children and families who have experiences like yours.

You can wear your own clothing most of the time and keep your special things with you.

You can talk or play with people who know how to help when you have questions or problems.

You can ask to be moved to another room if you are uncomfortable or unhappy.

Care that respects your need to grow, play, and learn.

We will consider all your interests and needs, not just those related to your illness or disability.

You have the right to rest, to play, and to learn. We will make sure that you have places and times for the things children your age need to grow and learn.

Making Choices and Decisions

Your ideas and feelings about how you want to be cared for are important.

You can tell us how we can help you feel more comfortable.

You can tell us how you want to take part in your care.

You can make choices whenever possible.

Sometimes you can decide when and where you get your treatments.

Source: BayState Medical Center. Used with permission.

Reporters and editors naturally write about their own experiences. Helen Lippman, executive editor of *Business & Health*, wrote a column about her attempts to obtain advice from physicians. In each example cited, her physicians gave her one-sentence answers instead of exploring how much she wanted to know. After Lippman reviewed the National Institutes of Health recommendation that women in their forties talk with their physician about whether to have yearly mammograms, she wrote, "The discrepancy between recommendation and reality suggests that the NIH experts don't know what it's like to be a layperson seeking medical advice from providers seeing patients on the run" (Lippman, 1997, p. 6). Lippman offered these suggestions to physicians for more effective communication with patients:

• Ask what the patient knows and feels.

• Review family history before responding.

• Offer educational materials to help patients learn more.

The *Wall Street Journal* published a story about a writer's attempt to select a new physician. After consulting a how-to guide on the subject, R. Langreth (1997, p. R4) reportedly found "receptionists who get annoyed by a simple inquiry; doctors who keep cushy hours even a banker would envy; doctors who refuse even to pick up the phone. Marcus Welby, where are you?" (Which reminds me of the old joke: Marcus Welby was wonderful, but he only had to take care of one patient a week.) Langreth suggested that readers call prospective physicians' offices and ask how long it would take to obtain a routine appointment (one week or less was considered good) and how many patients the doctor sees in a day. (Here, fewer than twenty-five to thirty was considered good.) Langreth went on to describe responses he received after asking if he could speak with the doctor for a moment at a convenient time. "The doctor doesn't do interviews," said one. "That would be a free consultation," said another. "God forbid," was the writer's response. He ultimately selected the physician whose receptionist answered his questions without hesitation, promised a quick appointment, and got the physician to return his telephone call.

Howard Maron and Scott Hall of Seattle, Washington, are creating a new version of Dr. Welby—a personal physician, on-call anytime. They retired from their medical practice, then invited a select group of patients to pay $12,000 per year for their services as family doctors and medical advisers. The physicians will accompany patients on visits to specialists, travel to evaluate or supervise care for out-of-town clients, deliver prescriptions, and take care of medical billing and paperwork.

While the media make heroes and celebrities of frequently cited or quoted physicians, on occasion a reporter helps manage the expectations of patients who want "only the best." The *Wall Street Journal*'s "Health Journal" is a prime example. Marilyn Chase (1996, p. B1) advised readers that "academic brilliance and patient skills don't necessarily overlap." Waiting for appointments, spending less time than might be expected in a medical visit, and possibly being seen by an associate of the star were mentioned as possible downsides of being seen by a well-known physician.

At the other end of the spectrum are the horror stories that may cause some patients to be unduly apprehensive about receiving care. Witness the impact on the dental profession after the Acer case was reported. Speculation that a dentist might have transmitted the HIV virus to his patients created widespread fear about obtaining dental care. Media attention paid to the transmission of diseases has made standard precautions something patients expect to see in a "good" physician's office.

To reduce the anxiety created by such media coverage, let patients see that you are taking precautions for their benefit. Instead of walking into the exam room wearing gloves, let your patient see you putting gloves on. Make sure all staff members delivering patient care wash their hands between patients. Posting your infection control procedures in your examining rooms and then following those procedures will guarantee that your patients' expectations will be met.

Even fictional television reflects what is being discussed in the press, and such portrayals can make patients apprehensive. Analyze what the media are saying. Are patients more or less likely to turn to you for care as a result of what they are learning from media sources?

Virtually every consumer magazine contains health and medical information. Many articles seek to promote more effective communication between patient and physician. They advise patients to pose such questions as: "What procedures are you recommending for me and why?" "How many of these procedures have you performed in the last year?" "How much time can I take before choosing a course of treatment?" The widespread availability of medical information has resulted in an increasing number of knowledgeable and confident patients who want to use what they have learned to help them make treatment decisions.

William Keenan, M.D., of Williamsport, Pennsylvania, has found that

> Occasionally, you will come across the patient who uses his medical knowledge to play oneupmanship with the physician, but the majority of well-informed patients are informed because they took an interest in learning more about their own health. While such patients occasionally have more questions and can initially take more time during an office visit, they are much more likely to know what medicines they are taking, what the possible side effects are, and when it is appropriate to contact you. Such patients are also much more likely to understand the risks and benefits of screening tests and proposed treatments [William Keenan, telephone interview with the author, 1998].

What is your response when a patient arrives with a stack of study abstracts?

Managed Care

Where once patients selected their own physicians and hospitals and were predisposed to trust and respect them, today patients routinely call their managed care company before seeking routine and emergency care. With whom or what, then, is their primary relationship? Patients feel compromised because they have been routed into managed care plans. When patients feel that they have no choice but to "choose" you, it is much harder to win them over. Although corporate America and many healthy Americans are willing to trade off choice for lower expenses, they are unwilling to embrace controls on access to service. Stories about the negative aspects of managed care have resulted in increased patient anxiety. Patients not only fear that you do not like their managed care plan but also scrutinize your decisions and wonder if you are over- or undertreating them. Are physicians more interested in their patients' well-being or their reimbursement schedules? In an article for the *Boston Globe*, Carol Gentry (1995, p. 12), wrote, "Paying doctors to curtail care is a corrosive practice that eventually will destroy the trust that underlies the doctor-patient relationship. Even when doctors are thoroughly justified in saying 'no' to patient requests, they will be tarred with suspicion." One physician, Michael S. Victoroff of Colorado, developed a pledge for his patients that outlined what he would and would not do regardless of a patient's source of financing for care (Exhibit 4.2).

Patient expectations in a managed care environment would be more realistic if patients understood their benefit plans, but most do not. Employees receive Summary Plan Descriptions (SPDs) once a year. Very few people read them. Most do not even recall receiving them. Then when the patient receives an Explanation of Benefits (EOB) statement, you receive the inevitable call, "What do you mean it's not covered?"

Exhibit 4.2. A Promise to My Patients Concerning Financial Conflicts Related to Health Insurance.

As your physician, it's important to me that you know my feelings about the financial issues in our relationship. It's especially important that you understand how I deal with the ethical conflicts that may arise from insurance plans and other financial influences upon the decisions we make together.

My greatest wish as a doctor is that you judge my care to be the best possible, according to your personal standards. For this to happen, I need to earn your trust as an ethical person, as well as a skillful practitioner. I want you to know that, among the values that govern my practice, I make the following promises to you:

- I will treat you as a person, first and always, and not as a means of creating profits for me or anyone else.

- I will never deceive you about my motives or intentions. I will not withhold information I believe you should have when I recommend a plan of treatment. My advice will always consider first what is best for you as a person, regardless of its financial implications for you, your insurance company or anyone else, including myself.

- I believe in cost-conscious care as a secondary goal of a good health system. I will be sensitive to financial issues that affect you. I will help you discover the costs of treatments and assist you in finding the most effective uses of your money for the sake of your health. I will help you distinguish between decisions based on costs as opposed to other factors.

- Regardless of the payment arrangements between us, every treatment or recommendation that I provide will be based on my belief that it is in your best interest. I will not participate in any plan that offers me compensation so heavily weighted toward cost containment that it could create a temptation to place this factor above your welfare. Nor will I offer you treatments on a fee-for-service basis that are inappropriate or unnecessary, or at unreasonable fees.

- As an incentive to bear costs in mind, some insurance plans base a portion of payment to me upon their savings from services you do not use. Their intent is to reduce thoughtless and unnecessary treatments. However, I will disregard this incentive until we have considered all treatment options.

- Occasionally, a procedure that may have little hope of benefit or that may not normally be "covered" by your insurance might still be appropriate for you to consider. I will support you in asking your insurance plan to pay for any reasonable treatment, regardless of plan policy. And I may also encourage you to pay yourself for "uncovered" items that I believe offer valuable benefits not available under your plan. However, I will advise you against procedures that are wasteful, frivolous or irrational.

- If I foresee a conflict between your welfare and any policy, contract, guideline, standard or law, I will disclose it to you. In the presence of uncertainty, I will help you choose a course of action that recognizes your values. On medical issues, I will not place my personal interests above yours, nor will I cooperate with others in doing so.

- Finally, if I feel that you or anyone is contemplating a course of action that is not in your interest, I will advise you of this.

I participate in managed care plans because many people have no other access to medical insurance and because I believe that *well-managed* care is far superior to traditional, *"un-managed"* care. Whatever form your health coverage takes, I intend always to deal honorably with you, your insurance company and everyone else in the system.

Please let me know if at any time you have a concern about the completeness, accuracy or bias of any information you have received from me, my staff, or any consultant or organization to whom I have referred you.

Your doctor

Source: Michael S. Victoroff, M.D. Used with permission.

Patient Understanding of Benefits

Although you may not want to be in the financial planning business, providing benefit information when patients need it can be of great value for patients. Some practices advise patients to send the SPD to the practice when they receive it, and the practice keeps it on file for them. Be aware of the services available from managed care companies so that you can provide plan benefit information. Some insurers have developed fax-back programs to provide timely information about plan design to patients and physicians in their network. Neil Baum, a New Orleans urologist and marketing expert, offers his patients a video that explains benefit plans, coinsurance, deductibles, and covered services to them at the moment when they need the information.

Demand Management Services

Pressures to contain medical costs led to the development of demand-management services and systems that can help patients decide on the appropriate level of care they need. Telephone triage or advice programs provide immediate access to a health care professional, with little or no cost to the patient. Nurse advice lines teach patients about what they can expect during treatment. The nurses who staff advice lines find that patients often want to discuss issues that they feel uncomfortable introducing with their physicians, such as obtaining a second opinion, mental health, sexuality, and sexually transmitted diseases; patients also call because they have not understood what their physician told them.

Employers are selecting self-care programs for their employees in order to reduce health care costs and utilization. They want you to support their efforts to provide employees with self-care information. If your patient receives *HealthWise* or another health information guide, be sure that you and your staff are very familiar with its contents.

Demand-management tools are often created as guidelines that clarify, in lay terms and from the patient's perspective, what will happen next. Whether the tool is a telephone decision-support service, a self-help handbook, or a support group, patients receive information that helps them understand their options and their eventual disease course. These services can have a significant impact on the patient's perceived need for various types of medical care.

> **Successful organizations convince patients that where other organizations have problems, they do not.**

The Positive Side of Managed Care

Successful organizations convince patients that where other organizations have problems, they do not. If you were a patient fed up with listening to the complaints of doctors about managed care, would you be inclined to consider the physician who wrote this letter to his local newspaper (Nedelman, 1996, p. 14)?

> *To the Editor:*
>
> *I have been practicing primary care medicine for 30 years and during this time have devoted my energies to preventive health care as well as the treatment of acute and chronic illness.*
>
> *Enter managed health care and now for the first time primary care physicians are being recognized as a sound investment in controlling medical costs.*
>
> *Physicians are being "graded" on the quality of their care by the HMO. Results of patient surveys regarding waiting time, courtesy of office staff and understanding physician instructions are being reported to the physician. HMOs in turn are able to report to physicians information such as percentage of yearly mammograms performed in their female population between ages 50 and 65, the number of adults whose cholesterol has been determined within the past five years and other indicators of preventive care that primary care physicians have always thought they have done a superb job. Surprisingly, for many physicians the results are not always as*

good as one might suspect and physicians now have new insight and information with which to energize their practice and provide a better and more comprehensive health care plan for the patient.

I believe that managed care with few exceptions has been an advocate of the consumer. Physicians are now more responsible for the health of their patients and must go that extra step to provide the immunizations, cholesterol, PSA, mammograms, etc. necessary for good health maintenance.

Early detection of disease has proven to be cost effective and HMOs are in the forefront requiring a higher level of care for patients from their primary care physician. The standards of HMOs benefit primarily one individual—the consumer.

Philip B. Nedelman M.D.
Braintree Family Physician, Inc.
Braintree, MA

•   •   •   •   •   •   •

Your concern for your patient's best interest can counteract any unrealistic expectations created by advertising, the media, and managed care. Managing expectations is less of a challenge when you are your patient's most credible resource for advice regarding his needs, beliefs, and preferences.

5

First Impressions

*Given two equally competent physicians, pick the one
with a smile and optimistic disposition.*

Nicholas Wade*

W hen a new patient calls and visits your organization for the
first time, he will decide whether your practice can give him
what he needs. Lawyers often coach their clients for hours on their
appearance in the courtroom. They invest the time because they
know that at least some of the jury members will decide the case
based on their initial impressions of the plaintiff and the defendant.
First impressions are important because people do act on them.
Have you ever walked into a restaurant and walked right out without being seated? Your first impression, based on your initial scan or
assessment of what's important to you, convinced you that the
restaurant would not provide what you were looking for.

Anxiety of the Uninitiated

Patients visiting your practice for the first time, particularly those
who have selected you from a managed care directory or the yellow
pages, may not have any idea of what to expect. They don't know

you, your system, what you stand for, or your reputation. Yet they want you to be someone they can trust. Lack of information about what to expect creates anxiety. Will he be treated courteously or with indifference? Are the people in the practice competent and reliable? Should he knock on that unfriendly glass partition and interrupt the receptionist? Or should he just take a seat and wait to be called? Will he be asked for the co-pay before or after he sees the physician? The patient is often clueless about what he's supposed to do.

Think for a moment about times when you have joined a new gym or visited a hair salon for the first time. If someone took the time to show your where to put your coat, introduced you to the owner, and showed you the features of the organization, you probably felt a lot more comfortable about returning. The same is true for a first-time visitor to your practice. Giving a tour, showing the sterilization equipment, and introducing staff members are all ways of reducing the anxiety of the uninitiated.

What would it be like for the anxious patient to receive a call from your practice prior to the first visit to introduce the organization, ask questions about his preferences, and send information in response to his identified needs?

Greeting Patients

The first sixty seconds of every encounter are critical to its success. I had a wonderful dentist. He was so good that I convinced my mother to become his patient even though she lived two hundred miles away. When he died unexpectedly, we each had difficulty finding a new dentist. One day, I asked, "Mom, why was he so special?"

"I think it was the way Denise [the receptionist] was always so happy to see me," she answered. She was right. The experience of enjoying the dental visit had everything to do with the receptionist's welcoming attitude.

Patients equate your ability to provide quality care and service with how knowledgeable and kind everyone in your practice is, beginning with the receptionist. As nice as your reception area may be, it means nothing if the patient is not acknowledged warmly when he arrives. The receptionist should not wait for patients to speak first. If the receptionist is having a personal conversation on the telephone and does not make eye contact or speak with the patient, no words have been exchanged. But the patient has received a message all the same, and it goes something like this: "I don't care who you are or what your problem is. I don't care about this practice or its patients. You can wait." A receptionist who is speaking to someone on the telephone as a patient arrives can still smile warmly. Assigning too many duties to a receptionist can interfere with the important responsibility of making patients feel welcome and comfortable. Patients should not be asked to state the purpose of their visit if other patients will overhear what is being said.

At the Williamsport Hospital in Williamsport, Pennsylvania, administrators found that although the encounters between the emergency department physician and the patient and between the emergency department nurse and the patient were important, it was the encounter between the emergency department *reception-ist* and the patient that was most important (Mannello, 1995). Improving that experience improved satisfaction ratings by emergency department patients dramatically.

Although the receptionist creates the initial expectations, each member of the practice must seek to establish immediate rapport with patients. Fostering a sense of trust and satisfaction should be a priority. Everything you say and do during the first moments of your encounter will increase or decrease rapport with the patient. How can you convey a welcoming attitude? Prepare for the visit by reminding yourself that making your patient feel welcome is important. Review the patient's chart in advance. Be the first to say hello, using the patient's name. You have heard all this before, but are you doing it? Use the same skills you use in social situations: introductions, shaking hands, speaking at the same physical level whenever possible. Try to avoid having physical barriers between you and the patient when you first meet him. Even holding the patient's chart against your chest can create a type of wall between the two of you. Parents often praise physicians and staff for speaking first to their child and for directing questions to the child whenever appropriate.

The Impression You Make

To make a good first impression is an opportunity that will never come again. When a physician appears annoyed, impatient, indignant, or condescending in a court appearance, her attorney has to spend as much time changing jury perceptions as she does on the merits of the case. When you appear rushed or indifferent or condescending to patients during a first visit, you too will have to invest significant time in changing those initial perceptions.

In a study of more than a thousand complaint letters from dissatisfied patients in a Michigan managed care plan (Beckman, Markakis, Suchman, and Frankel, 1994), 90 percent of the complaints focused on the communication style of the patient's physician. "The most common complaint had to do with a lack of compassion on the physician's part," said Richard Frankel of the University of Rochester Medical School. "Patients would complain their physician never looked at them during the entire encounter, made them feel humiliated or used medical jargon that left them confused."

Terrence Rynne, president of Rynne Marketing Group, talks about "cues to quality"—the cues patients use to link features to the benefits of a product or service. During the first moment of an encounter, potential customers are at their most alert, seeking information and assessing cues. As an example, Rynne states that a patient may perceive the benefit of being well cared for by the feature of the physician's being attentive. The cue might be any or all of the following:

- Having an open, friendly face
- Looking the patient in the eye

- Addressing the patient by name

- Entering the exam room after reviewing the patient's chart

- Sitting down at eye level

- Greeting with a handshake

"Controlling the cues can shape positive judgments into purchases and satisfaction. Anyone looking to increase market share had better squarely focus on the moments when individual purchase decisions are made, and get them right," says Rynne (personal communication, 1998). Patients may not be experts, but they must make a decision. Therefore they use and rely on their own cues to quality.

Reception Area

A focus-group participant said one day: "Everyone wants the same things. They want the doctor's office to be clean and the people there to be friendly." Cleanliness is extremely important. People seek to confirm their first impressions. The patient who spots coffee stains on a chair in the reception area will be checking to see if your examination room equipment is dirty too. You may have experienced this yourself when you visited the lavatory before eating a meal at a restaurant. If the bathroom wasn't clean, how did you feel about eating the food? There's an old saying, "The guest sees more in an hour than the host sees in a year." Take a hard look at the cleanliness of your reception area. Perhaps it has been overlooked occasionally in the interest of keeping patient care areas spotless.

For some patients, the newness of your reception area reflects your commitment to state-of-the-art medical care. The *Wall Street Journal* reported on a study of patient reactions to doctors' offices that indicated that people do change physicians because they feel uneasy in the office. "I don't think people doctor-jump because they don't like the doctor but because they don't like the context," said psychologist Kate Altork, who was interviewed for the article (Bannon, 1997, p. B1). She found that patients preferred amenities and features such as plants, tissues, water coolers, telephones, and bowls of candy in the reception area; flowers in the lobby; windows in examining rooms; and dressing gowns that wrap around the entire body.

Your reception area can be used to make connections with patients. One practice created a videotape of every employee talking about himself or herself and how they perform their jobs. Hang photographs of your favorite (but not too upscale) vacation spot to give you a connection with your patients who love the same place. Hanging beautiful photographs of the town in which your practice is located shows pride in your community. An aerial photograph of the community can be very interesting. Perhaps you want patients to understand that you have personal as well as professional responsibilities. One way to convey this is to have a few current family photographs in the reception area. Unless you practice in an affluent area, these should not be family vacation pictures from exotic locations but rather school photos or candids. Consider your patient population when deciding on family photographs as part of the decor. Middle-aged and older women react negatively to male physicians who display photos of teenage daughters while the wife's photograph is nowhere to be seen. If you are a psychiatrist who specializes in caring for couples dealing with infertility, think twice about prominently displaying the giant photo of your eight children helping you trim the Christmas tree.

Monitor the reading materials in your reception area. Airlines don't run movies that involve plane crashes, and you should think twice about displaying magazines with such headlines as "How I Made Millions Suing Doctors for Malpractice." As discussed in Chapter Four, the tremendous amount of medical information in consumer magazines also creates expectations for patients. For example, the October 1996 issue of Good Housekeeping included an article titled "Breast Exam: Is Your Doctor Doing It Right?" The subtitle: "Find Out What Too Many Doctors—Maybe Yours—Do Wrong." A patient who read that article while waiting for you to do a breast exam might wonder about your competence if you did not do the exam exactly as described, while the patient was lying down and again while she was sitting or standing. Being aware of articles in current issues of magazines can alert you to increased numbers of questions about certain medications or procedures.

Physicians who limit their magazine collections to their own interests create an impression that they are more interested in themselves than in their patients. Physicians who ask office staff to bring in magazines from home may be representing themselves as tightwads.

Some practices ask patients for permission to place their thank-you letters in an album in the reception area. Waiting patients get a positive idea of what to expect. Consider an "If I Can Do It, Anyone Can" bulletin board. Testimonials from patients about how they have modified health behaviors or learned to live successfully with their illnesses can be inspiring and comforting to new patients.

Telephone Communication

A person may form a first impression of your practice when he calls your practice for the first time. How are telephone calls answered? Are calls handled promptly and with empathy, or are they viewed as annoying interruptions in the day's routine? Impatience or annoyance does not help a telephone call proceed any faster or more smoothly.

Voice consultants say that callers begin to make relatively durable first impressions within six to twelve seconds of perceiving a sensory cue, such as tone, volume, enthusiasm, inflection, or speed of speech. Impressions can include what the person looks like, whether or not she is smiling, and her personality and intellectual ability. Patients often generalize their impressions to include the entire practice the speaker is representing. Ask staff members to treat each call as if the caller were a special friend.

If team members hesitate to answer the telephone, it may be because they are insecure about whether they can answer the caller's questions or about how to use the features of the telephone system. Does everyone in the practice know how to transfer a call? Don't be too sure.

People develop negative impressions when the telephone rings too long. When a caller receives a busy signal over several tries, he may form an impression that the practice is too busy to attend to his needs. An automatic answering system may also give the impression that you are too busy to handle any new patients.

Telephone lines should be open from 9:00 A.M. to 5:00 P.M. Mondays through Fridays. Review any patterns that may have developed solely for staff convenience. Giving calls to the answering service during the noon hour is an obstacle not only for new patients but for patients with urgent problems who must then have the service contact you. Just as some people call a customer service department before they buy a computer, some prospective patients check out your practice before signing up. Practices that busy-out all of the lines for several hours a day in order to "catch up" create considerable animosity among patients. This practice has become so common in some parts of the country that health advocates are advising parents to avoid pediatric practices that they cannot contact immediately. "If a practice can't handle its phones, forget it," prospective patients are being told.

Patients perceive quality problems when voice mail is confusing, when they spend a long time in a hold pattern, when they are not told that they are being transferred, when calls are not returned as promised, when incorrect or inadequate messages are taken, and when they perceive responses to be impolite or indifferent.

When patients call, they want individualized service and a pleasant, interactive experience. That's why people react so negatively to "Doctor's office, please hold." If you are in the habit of shouting, "It's me! Don't put me on hold!" when you call your practice, your systems need improving. ("Improvement" does *not* mean installing a private line for you and your staff to use.) Staff members at some practices provide information before putting a caller on hold. For example: "Dr. Stanley's office. There is one call ahead of you. Can you hold?"

Select a consistent opening that everyone agrees to use when answering the telephone. Consider such alternatives as these:

Thank you for calling the Norwood Medical Group.

Good morning, thank you for calling the Norwood Medical Group.

Good morning, Norwood Medical Group. This is Al Mastera. How may I help you?

If your practice is too busy for any of these openers, at least let the patient know that he has reached the right organization. "Norwood Medical Group" is more professional than "Doctor's office."

Listen to your staff speaking on the telephone. What are they saying, and how are they saying it? An incomplete or impolite response sends a message about your competence and your compassion. Because everyone is her own worst critic, it also can be helpful to tape-record your side of the conversation for an hour or so, then replay the tape and conduct a self-assessment.

Address Your Patient's Needs First

When someone calls your practice, find out what he needs before taking care of your own needs. Think about calls you place to catalogue companies. A typical call might go something like this:

Thank you for calling the GHI Catalogue. May I have the customer ID number from the back of your catalogue?

Thank you. May I have the source code that is printed next to the customer ID number? Thank you. What credit card will you be using today? Thank you. May I have the expiration date? Thank you. Is the card issued in your name? Thank you. May I have your name as it appears on the card, please. Thank you. And what is your daytime telephone number? And your address? Will we be shipping to this address? Thank you. What is the first item number? Oh, I'm sorry, we're out of stock on that item.

You're left feeling frustrated and, perhaps, slightly abused. When you call a company that excels in customer service, the call goes like this:

"Thank you for calling the World-Class Catalogue Company. This is Patricia. How may I help you?"

"I'd like to place an order for a flannel shirt and jeans."

"Thank you. What is the first item number?"

So find out what your patients want first. If your first priority is obtaining insurance information, you create an impression that you care more about the patient's insurance company than you do about the patient. So many people hate being asked for insurance information first that it just isn't worth doing it that way anymore. It is inconsistent to say, "Patients are our first concern," and then act as though the insurance company is more important.

What would you think if you called a store to order a gift certificate and the employee answering the telephone said, "Well, I'm not sure we do gift certificates, please hold." Would you have confidence that they wanted or were prepared to receive your business? Your practice generates the same feeling when the person answering the telephone can't tell a prospective patient which health plans you participate with. Everyone in the practice should have easy access to information for responding to the most commonly asked questions. When the person answering the telephone can't make an appointment for the patient, or when the person calling to request an appointment is kept on hold too long, you have access problems. And poor access means lower revenues for your practice.

Listen carefully for the caller's name at the beginning of the call. Most people answering a telephone focus on whether the call is for them or what the call is about. The most important aspect of the call is who is calling. Health care is a business based on intimate relationships: patients should never hear, "I'm sorry, what was your name again?" When you concentrate on learning the caller's name at the outset, you can use his name during the conversation to create a favorable impression.

Callers often say something during a conversation that you can quickly comment on to show your interest in them. For example, the patient who has to cancel his appointment might explain that his young child is home sick with the flu. Take a moment to say, "I hope Melissa is feeling better soon." A health care professional told me a story about calling obstetricians' offices to schedule appointments to meet the physicians before selecting one. When she called the first office, the receptionist ended the conversation with "Be sure to bring your insurance card with you." When she called the second office, the conversation ended this way: "Be sure to bring your insurance card with you, and congratulations." She chose the second practice and has referred other patients to it. "I just knew I would feel comfortable there," was her comment. Using a relationship builder takes very little time, costs nothing, and has high impact.

To minimize the risk of misunderstandings and unmet expectations, summarize what you and the caller have agreed to do as a result of the call. Let the patient know what will happen next and when. "Dr. Walker will telephone the prescription in to the Abbot Pharmacy in Oakland before 3:00 P.M. today." When appropriate, ask the patient to give the summary. "Would you like to repeat those directions back to me?"

At the conclusion of the call, you can create a favorable impression by asking the caller, "Is there anything else I can do for you today?" Most of the time there won't be, but callers will hang up with a sense that you are interested in their needs. When possible, let the caller hang up first.

The following list summarizes the keys to an effective telephone call:

1. Listen for the caller's name at the outset.

2. Use the caller's name at least once during your conversation.

3. Find out the caller's need first.

4. Use a relationship builder.

5. At the conclusion of the call, ask, "Is there anything else I can do for you today?"

Every person answering the telephone should be knowledgeable about the services you provide. A high school student who works part-time in a cardiology practice and who does not know what an angioplasty is can make that practice appear less credible. The same is often true of temporary staff. "I'm just a temp" is a response that says, "Don't expect anything of me. I may or may not be right, I'm only here for the day." How realistic is it for you to expect a temporary staff person without training to understand the capabilities and limitations of your organization? If you use temporary or per diem staff, you should definitely invest in scripting.

Scripting

In his book *Father, Son & Co.*, Thomas Watson Jr. (1990) described a technique that his father considered critically important to the development and success of IBM. Thomas Watson Sr. prepared scripts for his salesforce to use. The scripts, coupled with good training, ensured that salespeople would give correct, consistent information presented in its most favorable light. Most important, the scripted information was presented in terms of how it would benefit the potential client.

Scripting provides complete and accurate information as quickly as patients need it. Scripting is like giving staff the encyclopedia to your practice. The easiest way to implement scripting is to start with information provided over the telephone. You know that many of the calls received by your practice are repetitive. "Which health plans do you participate with?" "Can you give me directions to your office?" When the person answering the telephone call can't answer questions confidently, everyone's time is wasted: the patient may feel the need to call again to verify that the information he received was correct; the person answering the telephone has to interrupt someone else's work to obtain the information the patient needs. Scripts become a central reference source that enables staff to provide information even when key people are away from the practice. If your orientation process is adequate, a patient should not be able to tell the difference between an employee who has been with you a few weeks and one who has been with you for years. Scripting shortens the learning curve and can eliminate bad telephone habits. The time saved by having information immediately available can be spent communicating that information in an engaging and courteous manner. Even routine information can be delivered in a personal way.

> Scripting provides complete and accurate information as quickly as patients need it.

Team members may balk at the need for scripts, or object to being "told what to say." They may protest that using scripts results in comments that sound "canned." Remind them that most people use internal scripts—ways that they have responded to a question or situation in the past. The problem with internal scripts is that they are often inconsistent, and inconsistency in presenting information to patients can lead to miscommunication, failure to follow through, and an adverse outcome. Time is wasted when patients feel that reliable information can only be obtained from the physician or a particular staff member. Formalizing a script helps everyone in the practice present information to patients in a positive manner, focusing on the benefit to the patient whenever possible.

Most people want to do the right thing, if they know what the right thing is. Scripting helps organizations provide the correct information. For example, a person new to an area telephoned several medical practices and asked if she could visit the office to meet the doctor. The responses were varied, with the majority of staffers replying, "I don't know, I'll have to check," or, "Please hold."

In one case the receptionist said, "Do you mean that you just want to come in and look at the office?"

"Yes," said the caller.

"Miss, that's not possible. You can make an appointment for a consultation, but you can't just come in. We don't have free visits here."

In another call, the receptionist responded, "Oh, we'd be pleased to have you visit our practice. Let's look at our schedules and find a convenient time for you and the doctor to meet." In both of these latter cases, the staff member answering the telephone may have been providing the exact message the physician wanted patients to hear. Then again, maybe not.

You can follow these steps to develop scripting for your practice:

1. For one week, ask every member of the team to keep a log of all the questions they receive over the telephone. Patients may be asking about the names and specialties of clinicians, the waiting time to obtain an appointment, or the number of similar conditions treated by the physicians in the practice. Asking staff to note their answers would be helpful, but having them do this may decrease the amount of information you receive, as people are reluctant to write down the questions and answers (Q & A) if they are uncertain about the accuracy of the response they gave.

2. Brainstorm with your leadership team to develop suggested responses to the questions. Consider how the responses can be used to create positive expectations for patients. For example, when writing down the directions to the practice, include

a description about the building or location that will help the caller find the address more easily and think favorably about coming to see you.

3. Review the Q & A with staff for accuracy and to identify areas in which responses could be improved.

4. Make the Q & A available to everyone.

Messages

Misunderstandings develop when information is improperly conveyed. What constitutes an emergency? How should such calls be handled? What symptoms require the immediate attention of a physician or other clinician? Every practice should select a specific form to be used by every person who takes messages. First, find out what the caller needs. Then obtain the other information needed to complete the form. Determine how soon the caller needs an answer. Commit to what can be delivered or present other options. Repeat key information to make sure it has been recorded accurately.

The following is an example of response to a nonurgent request: "Thank you, Mrs. Jones. I'll give Dr. Kaoud your message and ask her to renew your prescription for Claritin at the DeBello Pharmacy on Main Street. I'll call you tomorrow at 555-3456 to let you know that this has been done. May I leave a message on your answering machine if you are unavailable? Is there anything else I can do for you this morning?"

What impressions do your messages leave with patients? Ask each staff member to leave a message on her home answering machine. When she returns home in the evening, she can listen and consider whether she would like hearing the message as a patient. One staff member heard herself saying, "You must call us; it's very important," and realized that the patient would be anxious because the practice was closed for the evening. She vowed to give more information when leaving messages for patients. You can use voice messaging systems that allow patients to call in at their convenience for confidential test results and follow-up advice.

Voice Mail

Use technology to draw patients to you rather than drive them away. Do not purchase equipment that prevents callers from leaving as long a message as they wish. Do not force first-time callers to use voice mail. Instead, review the voice mail system with a new patient during the initial visit. Help patients feel comfortable using voice mail. Without education, patients may feel that your goal is to automate every area of the organization so that staff are not "bothered" by calls from patients. Do not screen callers with a lengthy list of options. Your system should allow callers to opt out immediately for emergencies and to opt out for a live person at any time. (There is a cartoon that shows a woman listening to a voice mail menu and hearing, "And for relief from this list of options, please hang up the phone.")

Ask a few patients to test your scripts for you before you implement them. Patients become frustrated when the voice mail options have nothing to do with the reasons they call. Test your voice mail options with patients often and listen to the reasons they give when they opt out to your staff. One practice included a reference to "the P.A.," who was the new clinician in the organization. A caller opted out to ask what Pennsylvania had to do with anything.

There are ways to personalize voice mail. Although the menu options should stay the same, team members can update their own messages each day. By including the date, an idea of the person's schedule, and a friendly tone of voice, technology can still be personal. Always end the outgoing voice mail message with a thank you. Frequent callers appreciate knowing how to bypass the message if they want to. Many systems allow callers to press 1 when the message begins so that they can go straight to the beep. Try to limit the number of options to four or fewer. The most frequently requested services should have the earliest prompts. For example, prescription refills might be "press 2," whereas questions about billing statements would be "press 4."

Providing a written key to the prompts and function of each prompt is helpful for patients, particularly older patients. One practice created a wallet-size card that listed both the menu options and the information the patient would need before placing the call, such as the name and telephone number of the pharmacy.

When you are connecting a patient to voice mail, it takes only a few seconds to explain to the patient that the person may not be at her desk and that the patient should leave a message so that the person can hear the message in the patient's own words. Also, ask the caller to leave a detailed message. This can save you considerable time. Voice mail does have the advantage of letting you hear patients give you their exact message, not one filtered by the message taker.

Monitor your patients' satisfaction with your voice mail system. Because of customer dissatisfaction, the Keena Manufacturing Corporation in Brunswick, Maine, eliminated voice mail (Epstein, 1997), and it trained customer service representatives to ask about the weather or vacations or a topic of interest to callers—something voice mail can't do.

It's often said that voice mail can be efficient or efficiently frustrating. What do your patients think about your system?

Speaker Telephones

This should really go without saying, but do not allow anyone in the practice to use a speaker telephone for conversations with patients. This is a prime example of technology pushing people away.

Answering Services

Your answering service may be open for business more hours than you are. Sometimes patients understand that they have reached an answering service; other times they don't. When a patient reaches the service but believes he has reached the office, his expectations are unlikely to be met—that is, unless you have a service that books appointments, resolves billing questions, and refills prescriptions for you.

The answering service is handling confidential and critically important information. Call your service regularly to see if your call is handled properly. Help the service help your patients by preparing specific guidelines on how you want calls to be handled. Keep the answering service apprised of events you are hosting or participating in. Send an annual photograph of your staff, identifying each person so that answering service personnel can visualize the people for whom they are taking calls. As with all vendors, positive relationships with your answering service personnel can generate positive word of mouth.

For after-hours coverage, have a system that works. Many patients react negatively to answering messages that say, "If this is an emergency, call Dr. Sussman's pager at 928-555-6321. When you hear three beeps, key in your number, push the pound key and hang up. Dr. Sussman will call you back." If you have decided on a system like this, it is critical that you teach patients how to feel comfortable with it before they leave the office. "Can you give me two minutes to show you how the pager system works?" Some patients don't know that the pound key is the one on the lower right corner of the telephone keypad.

If you have a coverage arrangement with another practice, always check to make sure that they have not signed out to *another* practice. These indirect coverage arrangements create uncertainty for the patient and the covering physician that diminishes the patient's confidence and trust in you.

Signage

Signage in your practice creates impressions. Do you have signs that help patients find your practice? The front door to your practice should be conspicuous to anyone seeking to visit you. Are there enough signs? Are they clear? A sign on the front door that reads, "Please come in," can be welcoming, but it doesn't work if you have a glass door that you lock during the lunch hour while staff members eat at their desks.

The best signs help patients understand how your practice works. A sign that reads, "Please give your name to the receptionist," can be confusing for patients who believe that the receptionist already knows their names. A better sign would be, "Please let our receptionist know that you are here."

A common sign in reception areas is, "Payment is expected at time of service, unless other arrangements have been made." Patients who have no intention of paying their bill at the time of their visit will assume that if other arrangements have ever been made, they can be made for them too. Patients who do pay at the time of the visit may wonder whether your preferred patients receive other arrangements. A better sign would be, "Payment is appreciated at the time of service."

A sign that tells patients which health plans you participate with reassures patients that you are still accepting their insurance. And the next time they have to select a health plan at work, they may be able to recall which plans you accept.

Review how many signs in the reception area relate to payment and insurance, as compared to the number that help patients feel comfortable and welcome. When too much emphasis is placed on payment, the receptionist might as well be saying, "The doctor will bill you now."

Too many signs plastered about can give the impression of a poorly organized practice, particularly if the signs are in different sizes, shapes, and typefaces.

Have you seen signs and bumper stickers that read, "The worst day at the beach is better than the best day at work?" What's the message? That you would be happier doing something else or doing what you do somewhere else. The worst days of those who enjoy what they do are better than the best days of those who do not.

Recently, I visited an academic medical center. I arrived at the reception area at 12:50 P.M. for a 1:00 P.M. appointment. The sign on the receptionist's desk said, "Be back from lunch at 12:45 P.M." When the receptionist arrived at 1:00 P.M., I introduced myself and said that I was there for a 1:00 P.M. X ray.

"Not on the schedule," she replied. I told her which department had made the appointment and that I was scheduled to see a specialist at 1:30, but that he couldn't see me without the X ray. "Well, you're not on the schedule," she replied, as if that would be the end of it.

Feeling my voice trembling, I said, "I realize that it is not your fault that I am not on the schedule, but I have traveled two hours to get here, and the doctor will be waiting to see me. Is there anything you can do?"

"I'll ask the technicians when they get back from lunch. Have a seat," was her reply.

She went off to do something, and I sat staring at the reception desk. Over her head, for all the world to see, was this sign:

I give 100 percent to my job

10 percent on Monday
25 percent on Tuesday
25 percent on Wednesday
25 percent on Thursday
 15 percent on Friday
100 percent

I was there on a Tuesday and receiving my full 25 percent. Signs like these can relieve staff stress but are best kept in private areas of the practice.

Forms

Registration forms can create negative impressions when original forms are copied to save money. Such forms are difficult to read and complete accurately, leading patients to believe that the information must not be very important. Simplify the wording on forms whenever possible, and consider the impression your wording creates for patients. One physician developed his own registration form that asked very detailed questions about the patient's financial status. If a patient asked why he needed so much information, the doctor would answer, "So that my collection agency can find you if you don't pay the bill." Impression: the doctor had to satisfy his collection agency's need for information because he had many unsatisfied patients who didn't pay their bills.

If you are taking care of older patients, invest in registration forms printed in a fourteen point or larger typeface, so that the patient is not embarrassed while completing the form.

First Impressions Test

Make two or more copies of the first impressions test provided in Exhibit 5.1. Complete one test yourself and ask one or more of your staff to complete duplicates. Less important than your score is the comparability of your responses. Where your answers differ, you have opportunities for improvement.

In the retail industry, there is a saying about customers: "Confuse them and lose them." When you compare your test answers with those of someone else in the practice, you may find that you provide service in very different ways. Such inconsistencies can lead to misunderstandings that when observed by patients, lessen their confidence in your organization.

Exhibit 5.1. First Impressions Test.

1. Is the practice easy to identify from the street?	YES	NO
2. Once inside the building, is it easy to find your office?	YES	NO
3. When you enter the office, is the air fresh?	YES	NO
4. If a glass partition separates the reception area and the receptionist, does the receptionist open it immediately when a visitor arrives? Answer yes if there is no partition.	YES	NO
5. Is the reception area furniture free of stains and tears?	YES	NO
6. Is there some individual seating in the reception area?	YES	NO
7. Are there current issues of at least eight different magazines?	YES	NO
8. Are patients greeted with a smile?	YES	NO
9. Do staff make eye contact with the patient?	YES	NO
10. Are first-time patients welcomed to the practice?	YES	NO
11. Does a form or a staff member ask the patient about the name he or she prefers to be called? Alternatively, are all adult patients addressed by their last names?	YES	NO
12. Are patients afforded privacy to explain why they are there?	YES	NO
13. Are patient names and records accessible to staff only?	YES	NO
14. Do staff orient patients about what will happen next?	YES	NO
15. Does the patient meet his or her physician before disrobing, giving a urine specimen, having blood pressure checked, and so on?	YES	NO
16. Is the practice free of flip and/or inappropriate signs?	YES	NO
17. Do patients see staff following standard precautions?	YES	NO
18. Do staff or physicians apologize for waits longer than five minutes?	YES	NO
19. Do staff members listen without interrupting?	YES	NO
20. Do physicians and staff appear to be happy in their positions?	YES	NO

Give your practice 5 points for every question answered yes.

85–100: WOW! 75–80: Some fine-tuning and you're exceptional.
60–70: Good, but improvement is possible. Below 60: Ouch!

Part II

Identifying Expectations

6

Listening Skills

Listening to customers is becoming a lost art. That's good news for people who still know how to do it.
Norm Brodsky

The best relationships in our lives are those in which we are treated with dignity and we treat others with dignity. You treat people with dignity when you show respect for them, and the sincerest form of respect is genuine listening. Most people in health care can easily identify at least one extremely competent physician who fails to build a successful practice because he believes that all it takes to be successful are good technical skills. Failing to recognize the value patients place on strong interpersonal skills, he is doomed to receive only the most difficult cases and patients. His own patients don't stay with him if they have an alternative. The one strategy that might salvage this physician's practice would be to develop effective listening skills. As author Denis Waitley (1995, p. 167) says, "Genuine listening can cure a remarkable range of supposedly intractable problems."

> The best relationships in our lives are those in which we are treated with dignity and we treat others with dignity.

Very Few Patients Tell You What They Want

Many patients think that a good physician will know what they need, just as too many people assume that if their spouse loved them, he or she would know what they want. Many couples are unhappy when one party doesn't intuitively live up to the other's expectations. In the same way, your patients may be dissatisfied because you have not lived up to their expectations, even though they haven't explicitly stated them to you.

You may rightfully believe that you know a great deal about your patient's presenting condition. But in every situation, there are numerous factors that you can't possibly be aware of unless you allow the patient to share his story. In the early stages of illness or the physician-patient relationship, patients often know the detailed circumstances of their illness better than you can. Understanding the complexity of the patient's story is important if you do not want to miss information that will prevent you from oversimplifying the story to fit your presumed diagnosis. One specialist told me that he could diagnose a given condition within sixty seconds of meeting a patient. When he made those instant diagnoses, he found that patients felt obligated to tell their story several times, to make sure he really understood them. Or they sought a second opinion. He learned that when he listened to their stories and asked several questions and then made the diagnosis, his patients felt far more confident about his diagnostic skills.

Three Steps to Effective Listening

There are three steps to effective listening: listening without interruption, obtaining clarification and acceptance, and responding.

Listening Without Interruption

Listening to patients is a bonding experience. Your patients may have few opportunities, outside of therapy, to tell their stories.

Being interested in what your patient has to say is important, but you should also *appear* interested. Look at the patient more than at the chart. If you review the chart prior to your meeting, you won't have the "interruption" of glancing at the chart while your patient speaks.

Look as though you are paying attention. When you are speaking, how does another person let you know that she is interested in what you are saying? Think of a time when you met someone who seemed very interested in you (perhaps a first date). How did that person let you know that he was genuinely paying attention? He might have

- Leaned toward you

- Maintained eye contact

- Asked questions about what you were saying

- Smiled, nodded, or used other facial expressions to show interest

- Agreed with something you said

- Tried to understand how you felt about what you were saying

Instead of responding quickly to the patient's first comment, use *continuers*, such as "I see," "Go on," "OK," or "I'm listening," to indicate your interest in what he has to say and to encourage the patient to provide more information.

Paraphrasing for Acceptance and Clarification

Sometimes we listen for what we expect to hear. There's an old story about the physician who entered the presurgical holding area and said to a young boy, "Are you Fred?" The boy thought the physician said, "Are you afraid?" and answered yes. The boy got the wrong surgery, and the physician got a distressing lawsuit.

When you take time to paraphrase their comments, your patients know that you have heard what they said and that you understand their sentiments. Paraphrasing is important because you won't always understand things the way the patient intended for them to be understood. And instead of saying, "Oh Doctor, I didn't mean that," the patient may let it pass in order to be agreeable or to avoid seeming unintelligent.

To paraphrase, begin with a statement like one of these:

So, you feel that . . .

From what I'm hearing, you want . . .

Let me be sure I understand your perspective.

I hear you saying . . .

Is this what you mean?

Let me see whether I follow you.

As I understand it . . .

Let's see if I understood you. You said . . .

Am I on target with what you meant?

Summarize the patient's major points. Pause between sentences to allow the patient to ask questions or correct what you have said. Then ask whether you have understood him correctly. Paraphrasing is a way to show empathy, to convey that you didn't just listen but that you understood. Oliver Wendell Holmes Sr. (1860) said, "A moment's insight is sometimes worth a life's experience." Paraphrasing is one of the easiest ways to gain insight about your patient's perspective.

Responding

When you are listening, limit your comments to short statements or, better yet, questions. Observation of patient styles can help you respond effectively. Sharon Moss, a USAirways customer service agent based in Nassau, Bahama Islands, noted in her company's customer magazine (Maxa, 1996, p. 112) that whereas vacationers are laid back, business travelers expect customer service to be quick and efficient. But for all customers, her motto is "Be quick to listen and slow to speak." At FedEx, a customer service representative expects that someone calling from New York will be brisk and to the point, whereas a caller from North Carolina will want some exchange of pleasantries. Nevertheless, the FedEx customer service rep will do a quick listening scan to determine what the pace and tone of the call should be in order to create a pleasant interaction for the customer.

While you are speaking, observe your patient's nonverbal responses, such as eye contact, quizzical glances, furrowed brows, and tense muscles. A patient who opens his mouth while you are speaking is indicating that he would like to interrupt what you are saying or get a word in edgewise.

Sometimes, when you want to make a quick connection you may not listen effectively. In an attempt to have something in common with a patient, you may respond with a connecting statement about yourself. So when a patient tells you that he's just returned from his vacation, instead of asking him about it you respond by telling him that you have just returned from vacation too. This is a particularly poor response when what you say can be interpreted as one-upmanship—if, for example, he went to the beach in the next town and you went to Europe. In an attempt to find something in common, many people say, "I know exactly how you feel. Listen to what happened to me . . ." If you relate most of what you hear to your own experience, your listening skills need improvement.

You might be tempted to proceed expediently and forgo asking questions when you are very busy. Asking questions does take additional time but can often save more time in the long run. When I would ask Lucille Lieberman, our health sciences librarian, to run a literature search for me, she would want to ask me several questions to find out exactly what I needed. Not wanting to take the time, I would say, "Lou, send me everything on the topic and I'll figure out what I need." It took me far too long to discover that when I took the time to answer her questions, she could identify articles that gave me specifically what I needed, often saving both of us hours of irrelevant research.

Learning to ask open-ended questions is a good start to effective listening. "Tell me, please, how we can improve our services for patients," is a better question than, "Do you have any suggestions for how we can improve our service?" Open-ended questions are helpful in obtaining information regarding expectations. What does the patient like and dislike? What has he already said yes or no to? What are his perceived needs? What are his unrecognized needs? Examples of open-ended questions include the following:

What questions do you have?

How can I help you today?

Can you tell me why you think this is happening?

That's interesting. Why do you think that is?

Would you like to add anything?

Some statements that patients make demand extra attention because they convey expectations:

I wish we could . . .

What I'm interested in is . . .

I thought that I would be . . .

I really need . . .

We want to . . .

I'm looking for . . .

We'd like to . . .

Affirm your interest with statements that encourage the patient to express his expectation(s):

I'd like to hear more about this.

Tell me more.

Can you add anything?

That's true.

Please start at the beginning.

Can you give me an example?

Asking a question or making an affirming comment in a softer, gentler tone of voice encourages patients to continue. This technique also encourages patients to ask questions and can prevent misunderstandings.

Avoid closed-ended questions, such as, "You don't need a wheelchair, do you?" or, "Don't you agree that it would be best to have the surgery?" These can result in nonverbal responses, such as a nod or shake of the head, a sigh or a roll of the eyes. Closed-ended questions do not give you as much of an opportunity to evaluate your patient's ability to comprehend information as open-ended questions do.

Ask your patient to define words that he repeats often. "What does that mean to you?" Subjective words may also need to be defined. "Soon" may mean three days to you but three hours to your patient.

Discover the Problem Your Patient Is Trying to Solve

Do not be so focused on giving a good answer that you don't really hear the patient's question. Perhaps your patient tells you about her menstrual cramps becoming irregular; you respond with your usual advice about menopause, but the patient's real concern is cancer.

Listen instead with the thought of asking a follow-up question. There's an old saying that the patient knows the answer. Psychiatrists are taught to respond to what the patient offers with another question, with the ultimate objective of helping the patient clarify what he wants.

Your patient's immediate concern might be, "What does the medication do?" "How sick am I going to get?" "What tests will I need to have?" "What should I do if these symptoms occur again?" Or the immediate concern might not be clinical at all. I was driving on a rainy highway two hundred miles from home when my car spun out of control and crashed. At the hospital, the physician explained that I needed sutures and asked my permission to have a resident treat me. Not wanting to be perceived as uncooperative or difficult, my response to the doctor was, "Fine." "Fine" is often *not* the best answer. In fact, I was saying to myself, "No, I'm not letting some resident practice on me!"

The resident appeared, introduced himself, told me what he was planning to do, and then said something that I have never forgotten: "Is there anything I can do to make you more comfortable before we begin?" It might have appeared that my problem was to find out the extent of my injuries. But in fact my immediate problem was that my skirt and stockings had been badly ripped in the crash, and I felt self-conscious lying on the stretcher. "Yes," I said. "I'd feel better if I had a sheet over my legs." Moments later, the sheet over my legs, I relaxed and thought to myself, "Wasn't I lucky to get such a great doctor." I knew full well at that moment that I couldn't judge his clinical competence, but his interest in what I felt I needed made him an excellent physician in my mind. (The wound healed beautifully.) Responding to your patient's immediate concern helps reduce anxiety and encourages him to listen to what you have to say.

A patient may be dissatisfied with physicians in general because they never understood what he really wanted. Barsky (1981) suggests that physicians listen for and ask about nonmedical issues, such as life stress, when patients present without some recent change of symptoms or disability. A physician could ask, "What changes have there been in your life recently?" or, "What led you to come in right now rather than last week or next week?"

Barriers to Effective Listening

Barriers to effective listening include not liking the speaker, lack of time or patience, physical barriers, hearing problems, speech impediments, not understanding the speaker's language or accent, and internal and external distractions.

Eliminating distractions helps you listen more effectively. You know that you are preoccupied when you have difficulty maintaining eye contact with someone. You are more likely to become distracted and misunderstand your patient when you are tired. When distractions such as overhead paging can't be removed, try looking at just one of the patient's eyes while you listen. (One consultant suggests practicing making eye contact with your dog if you suffer from an eye contact deficiency.) Sit up straight, keep your body open, and smile when appropriate.

Interruptions

Finish documentation or arrangements for other patients before meeting your next patient. If staff frequently break into patient visits with questions about your orders for prior patients, assess the quality of your instructions. Do not permit staff members to interrupt patient visits, except for true emergencies. You may have become immune to staff interruptions, but your patients have not.

One patient said of her evaluation by an orthopedic surgeon:

> This doctor was too busy. As he was looking at my X rays
> and giving me a diagnosis in his office, he had another
> patient on a telephone call. He kept telling the patient
> to wait while he spoke to me. Then he would go back to

the telephone conversation, while I was sitting there, and speak to the other patient. A year later, another surgeon looked at my X rays and told me that I had a ruptured disc. Dr. Telephone's own report stated this, but he never discussed it with me, probably because he was trying to do two things at once. I was angry that I spent a year in pain when surgery was indicated, but even angrier about the way he treated me.

Internal Distractions

Because you can hear more words per minute than most people can speak, your mind is prone to wander. If you are preoccupied about something or someone, your patient will sense it. Inner distractions prevent effective listening. Physicians who feel pressured to achieve a certain level of productivity may feel uncomfortable about taking extra time to listen. A physician who has been chastised or financially penalized because she has not persuaded enough patients to have mammograms may focus narrowly on the need to recommend the exam and miss other cues or important information.

When you are stressed, you are more likely to be distracted. If family members, friends, or colleagues say, "Please look at me when I'm talking to you," or, "You never listen to me," let those comments serve as a red flag that stress is getting in the way of effective listening.

Try this exercise with your staff:

1. Team up in pairs.

2. Person A speaks to person B for three minutes about something he or she is interested in (possible topics: restaurants, favorite foods, last vacation, children, pets, sports team).

3. Person B listens but does not make eye contact. Person B may write some notes, look around the room, clear her throat, drink water, wave to someone on another team, and so on.

4. At the end of three minutes, repeat the exercise so that Person B has an opportunity to speak while Person A practices "disinterested listening."

5. At the conclusion of the exercise, ask people to share what actions show lack of interest. Responses might include looking at a clock or watch, edging toward the door, and not responding to statements.

The benefit of this exercise is in learning how discouraging it can be to talk with someone who is distracted or trying to do two or more things at once.

There may be triggers that cause you to stop listening. One physician, for example, tried to end conversations quickly whenever someone told her she looked tired. Another physician launched a tirade whenever one of her patients mentioned managed care.

Judgmental Listening

When egos are at stake, you may respond in a judgmental manner, especially when the patient takes a position that is in opposition to something about which you feel strongly. Such responses as, "You thought what?" or, "How could you?" or, "Why didn't you?" may prevent you from learning useful information, if your patient is afraid that you will criticize or ridicule him.

When you are not on the same physical level as the patient, you may give an impression that you don't have time to listen. In hospitals, it is often said that two minutes sitting at the bedside is better than ten minutes standing in the doorway or fifteen minutes standing in the doorway with one's hand on the doorknob.

Another barrier to effective listening is moving too quickly from listening to your findings. Brief listening limits dialogue and can result in the frustrating experience of dealing with the patient who raises new issues during the closing moments of the visit.

When you do most of the talking, you may not realize that there has been premature closure of a discussion and that the patient's needs may not have been met. If doing most of the talking is one of your barriers, consider a strategy suggested by Greg Korneluk, chairman of the International Council for Quality Care in Boca Raton, Florida (personal communication, 1998). He recommends that arriving patients be given an index card on which to write the three questions they would like to have answered during the visit. The card reminds the physician to address a patient's chief concerns. One physician told me that a few of his managed care patients interpreted this to mean that they could ask only three questions. He changed the text on his cards to read, "Please write down the questions that are of greatest concern to you today."

BATHE Technique

Sometimes patients visit you with so many problems that you couldn't possibly resolve them all even if you had unlimited time and energy. In these cases listening can be frustrating and may sap your energy. The BATHE technique, developed by Stuart and Lieberman (1986) in their book *The Fifteen Minute Hour: Applied Psychotherapy for the Primary Care Physician*, is a valuable strategy for helping patients with extensive nonmedical concerns.

B   stands for BACKGROUND
"What is going on it your life?" will elicit the context of the patient's visit.

A   stands for AFFECT
"How do you feel about what is going on?" allows the patient to report his current feelings.

T   stands for TROUBLE
"What about the situation troubles you the most?" helps you and the patient focus on one aspect of the problem.

H   stands for HANDLING
"How are you handling that?" gives an assessment of how
the patient is functioning.

E   stands for EMPATHY
"That must be very difficult for you." You then reinforce
the patient's coping skills or suggest alternatives.

Tools That Support Listening

Joseph Wassersug (letter to the author, 1998) suggests that physicians write down the patient's chief complaint and underline it as a reminder to address that specific issue. Keep in mind that the patient's first complaint may not be what he regards as most important.

Documenting patient expectations provides a sense of direction and a baseline to evaluate whether you are meeting expectations. Delbanco (1992) suggests a seven-dimension patient review to facilitate this process:

1. Respect for the patient's values, preferences, and expressed needs

2. Communication and education

3. Coordination and integration of care

4. Physical comfort

5. Emotional support and alleviation of fears and anxieties

6. Involvement of family and friends

7. Continuity and transition

When meeting a new patient, speak about yourself briefly and concentrate on topics that will benefit the patient or on things that you have learned you have in common. For example, "I want to be a resource to you so that you can make the best decisions about your health, now and in the future. With that in mind, help me understand what's important about your health to you? Give me some perspective on what's important to you in your relationship with me as your physician."

When you ask for information, you then have to respond to it very specifically in order to avoid creating expectations where they didn't exist before. Be prepared to explain your views, responsibilities, and methods—again in terms of the benefit to the patient whenever possible. One of the goals of listening is to determine whether you and your patient have similar expectations for treatment and outcome. Patients whose expectations are significantly higher than yours may choose another physician if you fail to recognize and address your different perspectives.

* * * * * * *

Listening is the most important of communication skills. Like other skills, listening can be enhanced through study and training. Improving your listening skills is an investment in the health of both your patients and your practice.

7

Patient Feedback

*Most of us would rather be ruined by praise than
saved by criticism.*

Norman Vincent Peale

Patients are, in one sense, your product. You want to know
whether they feel better—physically, emotionally, or both—
after a visit with you. Perhaps you already know. After all, you
know your patients better than anyone, right? You talk with them
every time they visit, and they tell you everything is fine, don't
they? Obtaining patient feedback is the best way to find out whether
you did what you promised and whether your patients' expectations
were met.

You know that patient satisfaction is important. Why are patient
satisfaction surveys important? Because assumptions about what patients want should always be tested. United Parcel Service (UPS)
thought its customers wanted on-time delivery. What their customers really wanted was more interaction with drivers, in order to
ask for advice or simply chat (Champy, 1997). The IRS thought its
customers wanted prompt tax refunds. What taxpayers really wanted
was no contact with the IRS (Gore, 1996). Just as it did for UPS
and the IRS, satisfaction survey information can provide insights
to guide your practice. You need the ideas and perceptions of

patients who have been in your care to reveal gaps between your assumptions and your patients' expectations.

Well-designed surveys provide you with meaningful information that you can use to improve service or change perceptions. One obstetrician learned through the survey process that patients thought she was unconcerned about how long they had to wait. The receptionist would say to patients, "She'll be with you shortly. She's just having her lunch." In reality, the solo practitioner was wolfing down a sandwich in her office while reviewing records of patients she would be seeing during the afternoon. She never took time for a lunch break in the hospital cafeteria or anywhere else. Asking the receptionist to eliminate references to lunch was an easy fix that improved patient perceptions.

Feedback encourages patients to help you achieve your organizational goals. Survey results can be used for

- Identifying problems promptly

- Recognizing staff

- Identifying the characteristics of good service

- Creating an opportunity for customer contact

- Staff training

- A source of patient suggestions

- Management reports

- Measuring quality improvements

- Determining patient preferences and expectations

- Identifying changing patient expectations

A patient satisfaction survey identifies what patients want, such as health information, counseling, or other services. The information you gain can aid your strategic planning by helping you determine whether or not to offer new services. Survey information can tell you whether something is what your patients truly want or merely what you think they want.

Including a question about whether a staff member provided exceptional service or exceeded the patient's expectations gives you an opportunity to recognize staff members who provide that kind of service.

Why Are You Surveying Patients?

What will you do with the data you gather from patients? Are you interested in comparing your practice with others regionally and nationally? Or would you like to limit your analysis to measuring improvements in your own practice over time? Are you primarily interested in having favorable data to use in your marketing efforts? One company went so far as to send surveys to customers with the answers already filled in (Heskett and others, 1994). Customers altered the marks only if they disagreed with the company's self-selected favorable ratings. One hopes that you are most interested in obtaining the kind of information that can be used to make positive changes in your practice.

Consultants are fond of saying, "Data, data everywhere, but not a drop of information." The most important commitment you make is deciding that you will act on the feedback you receive. The key is to collect and consider information in an unbiased manner and then put it to use. Some practices make the mistake of sending out hundreds of surveys that no one has time to review, much less analyze and act on. Data are often months, even years old before they are shared with people who can use the information. At the very least, commit to sharing timely information with staff via newsletters, reports, and inservice educational

> The most important commitment you make is deciding that you will act on the feedback you receive.

programs. If your staff members do not read and use survey information, your reporting system is ineffective. Perhaps it needs to be simplified. For example, every employee of Winter Silks, a silk clothing catalogue, receives a top-ten list of positive and negative customer comments each month (Caggiano, 1997). Ask your staff members how they use survey information and how it might be presented so as to be more valuable to them.

Survey Design: Do It Yourself?

It's surprising that people who insist on accuracy in financial reports are willing to accept poorly reasoned data on their satisfaction surveys. They accept poorly constructed survey instruments because they fail to recognize that it is patient satisfaction, perceptions, loyalty, and retention that drive financial results.

Designing a patient satisfaction survey is not a ten-minute exercise. Choosing what to measure is not a simple task. Satisfaction measures can be the right answers to the wrong questions. How much data can you collect and analyze effectively? Which patients should be surveyed? Should you exclude patients seen on Mondays who might be sicker or might feel rushed because you squeezed them into your schedule? Should you over-sample patients forty-five years old and older to measure the satisfaction of heavier users of medical services? Should you survey only active patients—those that have been seen within the past year? Should you exclude new patients who have not been with you long enough to give a fair assessment? If you limit the number of responses for patients to choose, will you end up hearing only what you want to hear?

Properly designed surveys can identify issues about which patients tend to have expectations, such as how well physicians and other clinicians listen, whether patients are involved in decision making as much as they would like to be, whether the patient assesses his health as improved, and the degree to which patients are encouraged to ask questions. It is worth the investment of time and money to see that your survey instrument has validity.

Some companies use two types of surveys: statistical surveys, designed to measure changes in customer perceptions over time, and comment surveys, designed to gather customers' top-of-mind needs and preferences. In an attempt to learn both what physicians wanted to know and what patients wanted to tell them, one practice combined the two concepts, using the survey shown in Exhibit 7.1.

Exhibit 7.1. Satisfaction Survey.

1. How satisfied are you with the care and service you receive from our practice?
- O   Very satisfied
- O   Somewhat satisfied
- O   Somewhat dissatisfied
- O   Very dissatisfied

2. How likely are you to choose to return to our practice the next time you need medical care?
- O   Definitely will
- O   Probably will
- O   Probably will not
- O   Definitely will not

3. If a friend were looking for a physician, how likely is it that you would recommend our practice?
- O   Definitely would
- O   Probably would
- O   Probably wouldn't
- O   Definitely wouldn't

4. Please tell us how we can improve our services for you:

_____

_____

_____

_____

_____ Thank you.

_____

The physicians used the first three questions to measure patient satisfaction, projected patient retention, and willingness to recommend the practice to others. Providing only four choices for responses forced the patient to choose whether he was more or less satisfied. The last question permitted patients to make suggestions for improvement in the practice. When patients signed their names to the survey, the practice was able to track, by each level of satisfaction, whether the patients remained loyal to the practice or not. Although many survey experts might consider this a less than perfect survey, it has provided the practice with exactly the information it considers most valuable.

At the Williamsport Hospital in Williamsport, Pennsylvania, the outpatient survey asks, "Have you used the Williamsport Hospital services before? If yes, has the quality of the services improved, remained the same, or declined?" The responses help measure trends in patients' perceptions of the organization.

At Thomas Jefferson University Hospital in Philadelphia, patients are surveyed during their inpatient admission and again several months after discharge. This two-part analysis provides information on first and lasting impressions and on patient loyalty.

Some hotel surveys ask questions that are written to help customers know whether or not they were well served. For example, "Did the bellman offer to get you some ice?" is a question that tells guests that if the bellman did offer, he did what was expected and the guest should be satisfied. Your survey questions can be used in the same way to manage patient expectations by identifying what should happen during an office visit. For example:

Did the receptionist greet you by name?

Did the physician encourage you to ask questions?

Did the physician give you written information that explained your condition?

Did the business office representative offer to submit your insurance claim for you?

Such questions as, "How long did you wait to obtain an appointment?" or, "How much time did the doctor spend with you?" can reveal gaps between your perceptions and those of your patients.

In addition to asking about satisfaction, ask patients to rank how important different variables are to their overall satisfaction. For example, if you ask about the reception area and telephone access, you may discover that 20 percent of patients responding to your survey think that your reception area looks tired. Another 20 percent may give the opinion that they often reach a busy signal when they telephone you. However, if you also find out that they consider being able to contact your practice of higher importance than the furnishings in the reception area, you have useful information on which to base your plans for improvement. In this scenario, based on patient feedback, your capital dollars would be better spent on adding additional telephone lines.

Let patients know in advance that your practice conducts surveys so that they are not surprised when contacted. Patients are more likely to complete surveys when they know that their physician supports the request for information.

Surveys Issued by Other Organizations

Surveys developed and administered by external organizations have two main advantages: the questions have usually been tested for validity, and you are able to compare your practice's survey results with those of similar practices.

Obtain copies of surveys that are sent to your patients by managed care companies or employers. Be familiar with what questions they ask. Staff members should review all satisfaction surveys, whether internal or external, during orientation and again on a periodic basis.

Tell Me What I Want to Hear

The value of one-on-one conversation with patients cannot be overestimated. Sophisticated research should not substitute for interaction with patients. Talking with patients is a simple, low-cost way to gain information regarding your patient's specific expectations and needs.

Although patients are keen observers, direct questioning may not produce suggestions you can actually work with. Truly dissatisfied patients have probably already left your practice. (Surveying former patients is discussed in Chapter Sixteen.) Current patients may be reluctant to provide negative feedback because they depend on you for their well-being. If your questions come as a surprise, they may not have enough time to think through their responses. Hesitation in answering may indicate that the patient is reluctant to provide candid feedback. You might try gentle questions such as, "Can you suggest any ways for us to improve service?" instead of, "Do you have any complaints?"

One highly effective question you can ask patients is, "Was it what you expected?" You can use this question after an office procedure, childbirth, surgery, or referral to another physician or health care organization. The patient's perspective will give you useful information in setting his future expectations and those of other patients.

If you or someone in your practice makes follow-up telephone calls to patients, consider asking them about their satisfaction during the call. Some consultants advise contacting patients within thirty days of their first appointment to discuss their satisfaction. Because new patients are at greater risk of leaving the practice than established patients, this is a worthwhile strategy to consider.

Patient satisfaction can be assessed through the Internet, by telephone, comment cards, focus groups, mystery patients, advisory councils, and, of course, through mail surveys. Each method has advantages and disadvantages. For example, McDonald's uses its Web site to ask customers for feedback on their eating habits and preferences. In this case, the advantage is that the information is received in a low-cost, timely manner. The disadvantage is that people using e-mail expect a response within twenty-four hours; a commitment of staff resources is needed to meet that expectation.

Mail surveys are the most common form of assessing patient and customer satisfaction. People receive so many mail surveys that obtaining a useful response rate can be a challenge. See Exhibit 7.2 for a list of strategies to improve mail survey response rates.

Telephone Surveys: Call Me Anytime, Except During Dinner

Telephone surveys can annoy patients, particularly when they are scheduled between 4:00 and 8:00 P.M., a time that consultants choose because it's easier to reach people then. (Surveyors should be flexible and offer alternate times to call the patient back.) Telephone surveys have also been criticized because patients don't feel that their responses are anonymous. After all, the surveyor has the patient's name and telephone number and knows that he has received medical care. Using automatic dialing systems (the computer calls the number and connects the surveyor to the caller only after a person answers the telephone) diminishes the importance of the patient's information in the same way that a form letter creates a different impression than a personally addressed one. If you use a telephone survey service, insist on professional interviewers and monitoring of interviews. The surveyor should let the patient know how long the survey will take. You also want to receive verbatim patient comments, not just an analysis. Without knowing the verbatim comments about her lunch, the physician whose patients regarded her as indifferent about their waiting would not have been able to change patient perceptions.

Exhibit 7.2. Mail Surveys: Twenty Strategies to Increase Response Rates.

1. Provide a postage-paid envelope for return. Better yet, provide a postage-paid self-mailer that can be sealed by the respondent.

2. The survey or survey envelope should be noticeably different from "junk" mail.

3. The request for completion of the survey should clearly state why you seek the respondent's participation and why it is important.

4. Provide a personal response to patients who sign the survey form.

5. Respond to ideas and suggestions. Post changes on your practice bulletin board or in your practice newsletter.

6. The patient's physician can give the survey to the patient and ask him or her to complete it at a convenient time, stressing that the information is helpful to the practice. Resist the temptation to give surveys only to the patients you like. If the survey is mailed, a sincere written request from the physician should be included.

7. Address envelopes by hand and use first-class stamps.

8. Sign by hand the letter asking for a response.

9. Offer to share the results of the survey with those who respond. Some people view this as an incentive.

10. Provide incentives, such as memo pads or notes with your practice name and telephone number. If you use an incentive, patients should simply receive it without any effort on their part. Incentives that have a connection to your practice are more memorable. An ophthalmology practice gave travel sewing kits that contained prethreaded sewing needles. (Note: focus-group participants have indicated that a short and important health care survey will be completed without an incentive.)

11. Response rates are higher when surveys are easy to understand and quick to complete. Most people do not read survey instructions. Avoid using "skip" questions, such as, "If your answer is No, skip to Section 3 on page 3." If you can't avoid skip patterns, telephone surveys may be a better choice for you. Avoid questions with double negatives. Ask questions in the order of the patient's experience. For example, questions about registration procedures should be asked at the beginning of the survey, not in the middle or at the end.

12. Provide the name and telephone number of someone to contact if respondents have questions about the survey or its validity.

13. Make follow-up telephone calls to ask for completion.

14. Send an advance letter stressing the importance of the survey.

15. Sending the questionnaire a second time is a worthwhile though expensive undertaking. A typical response to a second questionnaire is 50 percent of the people who did not respond to the first questionnaire.

16. Adding color draws attention to a survey.

17. Asking for sensitive personal information, such as income, decreases response.

18. In general, the shorter the questionnaire, the better the response.

19. If you are conducting ongoing surveys (as opposed to working with randomly selected patients using a specific time period for responses), have the surveys available wherever patients spend time in your practice, such as the reception area, examination rooms, and the billing counter.

20. Make the questions interesting and perhaps entertaining.

Results can be biased by the interviewer, whether that person is from your organization or an external vendor. The patient may answer questions differently because of the sex, age, accent, or tone of voice of the caller. If questions are confusing to the patient, the interviewer may try to clarify the questions with her own understanding of the questions, which may be incorrect.

One advantage of a telephone survey is that if it is conducted within a week after care was provided, the patient probably has a strong recollection of his experience and will be more motivated to talk about it than he will be when he receives a survey some time later.

An advantage of using your own staff to make telephone calls is that patients may not feel as apprehensive about the confidentiality of their information. A staff member is also in a better position to provide information the patient requests during the call. If you do use your staff to survey patients by telephone, try to choose a member of the team who has not cared directly for the patient.

An alternative to telephoning patients is to ask them to call you. Recognizing that months-old data were an impediment to responsiveness, Cleveland's MetroHealth System teamed up with Sprint Healthcare Systems to create an interactive telephone survey (Serb, 1997). Patients call a toll-free number and respond to recorded questions, receiving fifteen minutes of free long-distance calls in return. Survey results are transmitted to system leaders within days.

Pillsbury uses an outside company, InTouch, for employees to call with anonymous comments and suggestions. Employees receive stickers, magnets, and wallet cards with the toll-free number so that they can call whenever they want to communicate something to top management. Comments received are transcribed verbatim, and the transcripts are sent to the CEO, who was amazed to discover how much genuinely useful information was received through this process. You might consider a similar program for your patients or employees.

Comment Cards

Having readily available comment cards gives patients an opportunity to share opinions with you whenever they want to. Gordon M. Bethune turned around Continental Airlines with a pledge to listen to employees and customers. In one of his in-flight magazine columns, "Listening to You," Bethune highlighted improvements that had been made as a result of customer feedback and asked customers, "If we need more help with our thinking, please let us know" (Bethune, 1995, p. 8). The postage-paid comment card was available just to the right of his column. Patients, like other customers, are often reluctant to ask for a comment card, so have them available at various locations throughout the practice and in communications you send to patients.

Some companies send packets to new customers to invite them, by providing postage-paid reply cards, to participate in meetings to learn more about the company and provide feedback on products and services.

Nordstrom sends a comment card with each order that reads, "We're listening. Thank you for your order. We hope it's everything you expected. We want you to know that we're counting on our customers to let us know how we're doing. On quality. On service. And on style. We welcome your comments, suggestions and requests. If you have a minute, please drop us a line." Other companies position their questions on the invoice that the customer returns with payment.

Some experts say that comment cards tend to be completed by the very satisfied or the very dissatisfied. However, patients who are very satisfied or very dissatisfied are the most likely to tell others their opinions, thus creating positive or negative word of mouth. Shouldn't you know what those opinions are?

Focus Groups

Some practices test their patient satisfaction surveys in a focus-group setting. This allows them to see where patients get stuck in responding to the questions and whether the issues addressed in the survey are the ones most important to their patients.

Focus groups get to the heart of how and why patients react positively or negatively to actions in your practice. It is those feelings that cause them to stay with you or leave the practice.

Comments by focus-group participants have been used to guide product development and advertising and even political campaigns. McDonald's "You deserve a break today" theme was developed after researchers heard participants say that they went to McDonald's because they wanted to take a break from a trying day or their normal routine. Today, focus groups are standard in all major political campaigns because politicians understand that, when analyzed correctly, the comments of participants accurately reflect public opinion. In the 1992 campaign between Bill Clinton and George Bush, Clinton was able to move voters past the issue of his alleged extramarital affair by adopting a strategy suggested by focus-group participants. Both he and Mrs. Clinton vaguely admitted to problems in the marriage and steadfastly maintained that any problems had been resolved. Focus groups thought that they should be forthright in meeting with the press but not engage in debate about the specific issue. This proved to be invaluable advice for the campaign.

Listening to patients' language gives good qualitative data. The following are examples of questions the focus-group facilitator could ask:

Tell me what an ideal visit to a doctor's office would be like.

What three or four words would you use to describe how you felt when you visited your doctor's office?

How did you feel when you were with your doctor?

How did your doctor make you feel about yourself?

What does your doctor's practice do that other practices do not?

How did you choose your doctor?

What do you like about your doctor's practice?

How could your doctor's practice improve service for you?

How would you describe your doctor's practice to a neighbor?

What would a doctor do to make you feel that you were well cared for?

In a focus group, people open up and say things that they would never say directly to the physician or a staff member. "What's it like to be a patient there?" the facilitator asked one group. A participant responded, "The doctor's very nice but what really gets me is how the receptionist greets all the men by name but barely has time for female patients." Another participant quickly agreed that she had noticed this too. The receptionist was surprised and dismayed when the feedback was shared with her. Because the practice cared mostly for women, she found it easier to remember who the male patients were. She promptly began to pay more attention to greeting female patients.

Some companies conduct focus groups with their difficult customers, feeling that if they can identify ways to satisfy those customers, they can take their business to a higher level of customer service.

A focus group of patients who are cared for in other practices can identify opportunities to differentiate your organization. You want to know what other practices are doing that might be shaping your patients' expectations. Conversely, you can find out what you do that your competition seemingly can't. Unmet expectations of patients who are not in your practice can help you decide on a marketing plan for a new service you are considering. When the owners of Nantucket Nectars, a beverage company, meet with groups, they distribute samples of Snapple, a competitor's product. Asking the groups to critique their competitor and its product helps Nantucket Nectars make improvements in its own beverages and advertising.

Mystery Patients

Retail chains use mystery shoppers and hotels use mystery guests to evaluate the experiences of their customers. A mystery patient will, at your request, call to make an appointment, sit in reception, ask staff members for something unusual, ask about another patient to see if confidentiality is protected, express a complaint, and evaluate how well clinical procedures are handled. If you have reason to believe that your patients are reluctant to be candid with you, you might consider the services of a mystery patient. Choose someone who has client references and who will make his evaluation after paying several visits to your practice.

To derive the most benefit from the results of this type of consultation, you will need specific information. The mystery patient's noting that a staff member didn't introduce herself to him is far more objective than merely citing, "Attitude needs improvement."

Prospective patients act like mystery shoppers when they stop by unannounced to see what your practice is like. These patients will judge the level of service and professionalism of your practice by the limited amount they are able to observe.

Group Research

Ask each of your staff members to ask three acquaintances the following questions:

1. Have you ever visited our practice (or organization)?
2. If yes, what was your experience like?
3. Have any of your friends ever mentioned our practice?
4. If yes, what did they say about it?

If staff members do this, it is likely that they will be asked some questions about your practice. So meet in advance to speak about what is unique about your practice and what you would like people to know about you that they might not already know.

Patient Advisory Council

A group of eight to ten patients, representing the kinds of patients you prefer to care for ("best patients") or comprising a representative mix of patients, can help advise you on how best to meet the needs of your patients. Best patients might be those who make the greatest number of referrals to your practice. However, patients you consider difficult can offer valuable perspective too. Council members can advise on patients' perceptions of the value of current and proposed programs, policies, and activities. They can give you information that helps you improve everything from registration to billing. They can review patient satisfaction data and recommend measures for improvement. They can identify new opportunities for you to uniquely position your practice in the marketplace. An orthopedic surgeon's council suggested sending postcards on injury prevention to runners who were preregistered for a marathon. The council members knew what information would be most helpful to the runners. Over time, their advice made the surgeon the physician of choice for athletes in that community.

Resist Taking Exception to Survey Findings

Suppose you have decided on a patient feedback method. The results come in, and you learn the following: "Your waiting room is tacky. The music is too loud. Your plants are dying. The front desk staff are rude. You have bad breath. You never ask me if I would like to have a nurse in the room while you examine me. You never tell me what's going on. You charge too much."

If your first response is to take exception, you are not alone. No one likes to hear that her baby is ugly. You may not believe what

you hear. One evening, I was presenting a seminar on patient satisfaction. A physician entered the room and told me that he already
knew everything there was to know on the subject. He took a seat
in the rear of the auditorium and sat there, arms crossed, with a
scowl on his face, throughout the program. Toward the end of the
evening, he raised his hand and asked a question: "Why do patients
always ask me if I'm having a bad day?" The laughter from the other
participants indicated that they knew the answer, but this physician
had ignored the evidence.

A common taking-exception response to unfavorable survey results is to challenge the survey methodology: The patients didn't report accurately. The research service didn't report accurately. They
didn't ask the right questions. The questions are flawed. The sample wasn't truly random. The national benchmarks have nothing to
do with our region. The patients in our practice are different.

You don't have to look far to find a critic of any survey instrument. Yes, you want to know that your survey methodology is
sound. But if you are going to ignore or take exception to the information you receive, why go to the trouble of asking for it?

In one study (Froelich and Welch, 1996), 360 ambulatory patients were given questionnaires about their expectations. Patients
said that receiving information about prevention, prognosis, diagnosis, and continuing care was important to them. The information
regarding their expectations was randomly given or not given to the
physicians treating the patients. Physicians who received the questionnaire information did not differ in their behavior from those
who didn't receive it. All of the physicians prescribed more medications than expected, and almost none discussed prevention or
prognosis. In the study, physician knowledge of patient expectations
did not increase the fulfillment of those expectations.

The only return on the investment you make to survey patients
is to *use* the information—to create change if the need for change is
indicated. One measure of the value of a patient satisfaction survey

program is whether or not it causes you to take action. What was the last operational decision you made on the basis of patient satisfaction survey results?

Please Get Back to Me

How many surveys have you completed? How many times have you ever heard back from an organization that asked you to complete their survey? World-class companies offer survey respondents an opportunity to be contacted by a company representative. For example, the respondent is asked, "Please give us your name and daytime telephone number if you would like someone from the practice to contact you" or, "If you would like a personal reply, please include your name and address." If your survey is conducted by telephone, you should ask for the best time to call, the home or work number for that time, and what issue the patient would like to address so that the appropriate person can return the call. If you choose to offer this benefit, be prepared to dedicate some staff time to this function.

◆ ◆ ◆ ◆ ◆ ◆ ◆

Whatever survey method you choose, ask yourself whether you would respond to a survey sent in the same manner. At what point are you irritating patients? Properly used, patient satisfaction surveys provide a unique opportunity for you to see yourself as your patient sees you. The value of the opportunity is in the action you take as a result of patient feedback. A Japanese proverb says it best: "To know and not to act is not to know at all."

Part III

Managing Patient Expectations

8

Moments of Truth

Excellence is to do a common thing in an uncommon
way.

Booker T. Washington

A moment of truth is the moment when your patient decides whether or not you are what you say you are. Every time you communicate with a patient, even if it is just for a few seconds, you give him an opportunity to evaluate how well you are meeting his expectations.

Companies all over the world analyze moments of truth to help employees understand the impact of their behavior on customers. The concept of the moment of truth was developed by Jan Carlzon (1987), the CEO whose turnaround of Scandinavian Airlines (SAS) made him a customer service legend. Carlzon realized that during each interaction between any SAS employee and a customer, an impression was created about his company. If the interaction, which might be as brief as fifteen seconds, was a good moment, his was a good airline. And if the moment was a bad moment, his was a bad airline. Thus each moment of truth was an opportunity for a customer to evaluate his relationship with the airline. Carlzon set out to define those moments of truth and the actions, statements, and characteristics that would make them good, bad, or exceptional in customers' minds.

Carlzon led the company with four guiding principles:

1. Everyone needs to know and feel that he is needed.
2. Everyone wants to be treated as an individual.
3. Giving someone the freedom to take responsibility releases resources that would otherwise remain concealed.
4. An individual without information cannot take responsibility, whereas an individual who is given information cannot help but take responsibility.

Using the moment of truth concept in your practice helps you identify the needs and the service requirements of your patient and define how you will meet those needs consistently. How do you use moments of truth in your practice? First, identify what the moments are. Second, describe those moments from the patient's point of view. What is a good moment? What is a bad moment? What is an exceptional moment?

Moment of truth exercises often begin with a nonmedical example, such as the experience of visiting a restaurant. How do you decide on a restaurant for a special dinner? Perhaps you had a prior experience there. If you hadn't, you may have heard something about it—a referral by word of mouth. You call the restaurant and experience a moment of truth that might be anything from impossible to difficult to gracious. If the person taking the reservation keeps you on hold or has the attitude that he is doing you a favor by giving you a table, you will form an impression. Then the evening for the special dinner arrives. You arrive at the restaurant on time. If your table won't be ready for fifteen minutes and you are told to wait in the bar, you form another impression. One can analyze the restaurant experience straight through dinner, dessert, and departure.

Contrast the way you treat guests in your home to the ways patients sometimes report being treated. When you invite friends to your home, you let them know that they are wanted. You give them clear directions about how to find your home. When they arrive at 7:00 P.M., you are ready to greet them. You introduce them to others who are present. You probably orient them to the surroundings ("This is the dining room"), even though it's far from necessary. You don't speak in a foreign language. You don't leave them sitting alone in the living room for forty minutes without telling them what's happening. If they ask for something, you would never say, "You're not our only guest, you know." You try to find common interests to talk about. When the visit is over, you thank them for coming. Are you treating patients the way you treat your guests at home?

It requires detailed attention to identify the processes patients go through and then to specify the behaviors you want from staff during each of those processes. The chart provided in Exhibit 8.1 is just a start. Connellan and Zemke (1993) suggest that each moment of truth be measured against five factors:

1. Reliability—your ability to deliver what you promise, accurately

2. Responsiveness—your willingness to help and the speed of your response

3. Assurance—your ability to convey and inspire trust and confidence

4. Empathy—your ability to convey caring and individualized attention

5. Tangibles—your appearance, as well as that of your staff, facility, and products

For example, imagine that a patient has called your organization to ask for directions. He needs to know how to reach your practice, and he expects that the directions will be explained clearly. You probably agree that when this caller hangs up the telephone, he should have a good understanding of where your practice is located.

Exhibit 8.1. Moments of Truth.

Moment	Bad	Good	Exceptional
Calling your organization			
Making an appointment			
Receiving directions			
Meeting the receptionist			
Waiting in reception			
Waiting in an exam room			
Meeting the clinician			
Giving a history			
Having an examination			
Having an invasive procedure			
Giving a lab specimen			
Receiving discharge instructions			
Leaving the organization			
Obtaining test results			
Receiving a bill			

A bad moment of truth might be that the person answering the phone is unsure about how to respond. Perhaps the staff member is new to the practice or uses public transportation. The caller may hear something like, "Well, you take Exit 7 and turn left at the end of the ramp. You go to the second set of lights and take a right. I don't know the name of the street but there's a bank on the corner. Then you go two blocks . . . or is it three blocks? Hold on a minute, I'll get Mary, she knows how to get here."

A good moment of truth would be that the directions have been written down and are readily available, so that any member of the team can give them to a caller. The staff person answering the telephone asks the caller where he is traveling from in order to give him specific instructions.

An exceptional moment of truth might be that the directions are available on your printed materials and Web site and that the staff member offers to fax or mail them to the patient. The directions include a positive reference to your location. "We're in a lovely Victorian building across the street from the city park. It's a white building with black shutters, and we have free parking behind the office." This moment of truth would score well with patients for being accurate, being responsive, inspiring confidence, providing individual attention, and having a positive appearance.

When identifying exceptional moments, even routine ones, concentrate on behaviors and attitudes that help reduce patient anxiety or manage patient expectations (or both). Strive to define *exceptional* as memorable. Making the moment memorable often results from using a relationship builder. For example, the patient who has called to ask for directions says, "Thanks for the directions. I'll be coming right after my interview for a new job." A relationship builder would be a reply such as, "Good luck, I hope it turns out well for you."

In seminars, as we do this exercise, I ask participants to think about how they would like patients to describe their practice. What would they like patients to say about the care and attention they received? Most people would like to be described as competent and caring. Competence can give the impression of officiousness to patients if caring is not equally emphasized during a moment of truth. Professionalism denotes courtesy, not pomposity. Sometimes I share these comments written by travel critic C. Petkanas (1995, p. 119:) "[The hosts] are not professional hoteliers, which occasionally shows. Monsieur greeted me when I arrived, then disappeared for 10 minutes to take a phone call. Worse, I struggled to my room with a suitcase and briefcase, while he led the way, carrying nothing." We then discuss similar observations we have made in health care settings, such as that of seeing employees get onto elevators before patients.

Greeting Patients

There are many moments of truth during a visit to a medical practice: undergoing tests, being examined, receiving the bill, scheduling the next appointment. One moment stands above the rest as the critical moment, and it is the one that should demand your immediate and complete attention when it occurs. That moment is the greeting you give when you first see your patient. Ruth Davidhizer (1995), dean and chair of health professions and nursing at Bethany College in Mishawaka, Indiana, called the introduction the first step in the therapeutic process. Chapter Five addressed strategies for effective greetings that create positive first impressions.

Exiting Your Encounter

Another critically important moment of truth is the conclusion of the patient's visit. Do not leave the room too quickly. Perhaps you have done all the right things: You have given your patient undivided attention for the first sixty seconds of your encounter. You have determined the patient's needs before addressing your own. You have been clear about who will do what after the visit. You

have encouraged questions and answered them. You have qualified
for "Physician of the Year." Then, in an attempt to keep on schedule, you dash out of the examining room, creating the final impression that you were rushed and that perhaps the patient did not
really get as much time as he needed. Instead, shake hands warmly
and provide positive reinforcement about your relationship by saying something like, "I'm glad you came in." The send-off should be
with as much cheerfulness and enthusiasm as you can muster. You
want your patient to end the visit feeling cared for and with a conviction that his decision to see you was a wise one. Leaving your
meeting slowly is an art, but then, so is medicine.

Ask everyone in the practice to try to connect with patients as
they leave. The Ritz Carlton hotels realized that without a warm
send-off, they were giving an impression that they took good care of
their guests until they got their money, and then—wham—they were
on to the next guest (Schneiderman, 1996). Taking a moment to acknowledge that the patient is leaving takes little time and no money.
"Thank you for coming to see us today, Mr. Byard." "It was nice to
see you today, Mrs. Yaro." "I'll look forward to seeing you again next
time, Mr. Rumilly." "Have a nice vacation, Mrs. Marrapodi."

A Name Is the Sweetest . . .

You must know your patients' names. There's no getting around it.
People want to trust their lives to people who know them. Using
the patient's name when you greet him says, "You've made the right
choice coming in today, because we're happy that you are part of
this practice. We like you." Do you remember the television sitcom
Cheers? Whenever the character Norm came into the bar, everyone
cried out his name. A place where everybody knows your name is a
place where you feel you belong. If your patient's name is difficult
to pronounce, ask the patient to say it slowly while you write it
down phonetically. Then repeat it to the patient.

A patient I'll call Mrs. Boodman described this experience at her fourth visit with her physician: "The doctor opened the door and with a big smile on her face asked, 'How do you feel since the miscarriage?' Well, I nearly fell off the table. I said 'I'm Mrs. Boodman.' Still she said, 'So, how are you?' I then replied, 'Doctor, I have not had a miscarriage. You have mistaken me for another patient.' I got off the table and left. I now have a physician who looks at the chart before she walks into the examining room and is well aware of the case at hand."

Make sure your patient records are accurate. How do you feel when you receive an important letter with your name misspelled? Errors in minor things can create doubt about your ability to handle important things.

Address patients appropriately. Call patients by their last names, unless they request that you use their first names. Some patients may feel that it is unfair for them to address you as "Doctor" while you call them by their first names. Many patients do not feel old enough to be called "Ma'am" or "Sir." It's an unwanted reminder of advancing age. Consider having a line on the registration form that asks patients for their preferred form of address. Or just ask the patient how he would like to be addressed.

Do not refer to your patients by their condition. At one practice, the receptionist said to the radiology technician, "You're here for the mammo? She's standing right there." You say that wouldn't happen in your practice? Well, it's happening in many practices, including some you might regard as first rate.

When you meet with your patient, give him your full attention. Your patient may feel ignored while you make a quick note in the previous patient's chart, give discharge or staff instructions, or say good-bye to that patient. Prepare for your meeting with your patient by looking at his chart ahead of time. A patient should not overhear you saying to a staff member, "Why is he here?" especially if you suggested the follow-up visit.

Help patients learn staff members' names by referring to them by name during your visit. Instead of saying "Stop at the desk with this form on your way out," say "Please give this form to Karen at the front desk as you leave." This is a no-cost strategy but an important one, as some patients will leave your practice if they don't feel comfortable with the office staff. You can help make connections between patients and staff members. Encourage new staff members to use the "Forrest Gump introduction" when they are introducing themselves to patients: give the first name twice. "Hello, I'm Forrest, Forrest Gump."

Most people want four things: to be right, to be listened to, to feel respected, and to belong. Responding to these needs forms the most basic of customer service strategies and a powerful one for those organizations that use it. One of the benefits of the moments of truth exercise is that it forces you to start doing the things you know you should be doing.

Other Moments

Almost every practice has business cards or appointment cards at the front desk. Offering and handing a patient your card is subtly different from simply making cards available, but speaks to a more equal relationship. If a patient offers you his business card, studying the card for a moment is a way of showing respect.

The staff in one practice decided that they could improve their routine for calling to remind a patient about an appointment. Instead of saying, "I'm calling to confirm your appointment," staff members say, "I'm looking forward to seeing you on . . ." They leave the telephone number for the practice in case the patient needs to contact them. They enunciate clearly and repeat the number.

Observing where patients have difficulties can help you define moments of truth. In discussing the "leaving the office" moment, staff members at one practice commented that a bad moment was when patients could not identify which door was the exit. Patients leaving often selected the wrong door and ended up in private offices or in the janitor's closet. Staff members defined exceptional as escorting patients to the correct door and labeling the door so that unaccompanied patients could find it easily. This practice hired a painter to create a "This Way Out" graphic for the door. The result: one potentially anxious moment eliminated.

Radiology technicians worked together to define moments of truth for women having mammograms. They defined a bad moment as one in which the patient was in pain and did not know how long the X ray would take. One of the items they agreed on was that after compressing the breast, they would ask the patient, "Can you tolerate this? It will take about three minutes." This strategy gave choice and control to patients and helped them tolerate the procedure better.

Would a pre-op telephone call be an exceptional moment of truth for your patients? Many patients expect a call the day after surgery from their surgeon or a member of the staff. How many patients expect a call from their surgeon the evening *before* surgery? My neurosurgeon, Dr. Carl Dila, telephoned me at home the evening before my back surgery. "I've been thinking about you and wondered if you have any last-minute questions," he said. I replied, "I've been thinking about you and hope that you're going to bed early tonight." The call lasted less than two minutes, but I will remember it always.

Test your findings with patients to see if you have developed meaningful criteria. Listening to patients' stories will help you understand what they consider critical to the success of a moment of truth. Customer service consultant and author Ron Zemke (1996) tells a story of hotel staff who analyzed a conference coffee break. The staff thought that coffee and the cleanliness of the table setting were most important. Guests thought coffee and accessible rest rooms and telephones were most important. "If we can so totally screw up the perception of a coffee break, think of what can happen when we're dealing with airplanes and automobiles," Zemke said. Or health care.

Financial Policy

When I ask doctors and patients what doctors are looking for in their relationships with patients, patients say that doctors want patients who pay their bills. Doctors say they want patients who trust them. Perhaps doctors want patients they can trust to pay their bills. Patients who trust you will be more satisfied, will look to you for information about new technologies and services, will make financial sacrifices to remain in your care, *and* will pay their bills.

If they can figure out your bill, that is. When patients don't understand the bills they receive from you, they have a tendency to postpone dealing with them or to ignore them altogether. Do your bills clearly explain whether or not insurance has been filed, what the insurance company has paid, and what balance the patient currently owes? Typical obstacles to paying bills are confusing terminology, uncertainty about whether insurance reimbursement has been received, not having a telephone number on the bill to call with questions, and a long lag time between services rendered and bill received. One way to encourage payment is to have a staff member call the patient a few days after he has received the bill to ask if he has any questions about it.

Prepare responses for the most common questions and complaints about billing procedures. This helps staff feel more confident about responding and prevents top-of-mind answers that may be inaccurate.

Gather a group of twelve-year-olds together and have them simplify a billing statement for you. The questions they ask and the suggestions they make will be very valuable in improving the clarity of your statements.

A financial policy can be very helpful in managing patient expectations. Make it available for patients without requiring them to ask for it.

Brochures

Brochures serve to answer many questions when they list office hours, practitioners and their specialties, available services, how to access the office, and financial policies. Review your printed materials to see that the typeface used is large enough for the age groups you serve. A common problem with brochures is that their authors sometimes create unrealistic expectations by promising more than the practice can deliver. For example, if it seems like a great idea to respond to patient telephone calls in an hour, the promise may be written into the brochure despite the fact that the practice has never been able to return every telephone call in an hour.

Going Forward

There are countless definitions of quality. Many organizations have adopted the definition that quality is meeting or exceeding customers' expectations 100 percent of the time. Others have defined quality as doing the right thing *right*. Moments of truth exercises help people know what the right thing is. They help you move beyond vague, subjective ideas, such as, "Answer the telephone courteously," to prescriptions, such as, "Answer the telephone within three rings." Developing operational definitions can prevent confusion and sometimes conflict.

Once you have defined your moments of truth, create visual reminders about the moments and recognize and reward staff members who make the exceptional moments happen.

The ways in which moments of truth are handled distinguishes one organization from another. People support what they help to create, and taking the time to engage your staff in analyzing moments of truth can result in some dramatic improvements in the kind of service you provide for patients.

9

Staff Strategies

*The deeper principle of human nature is the desire to
be appreciated.*

William James

The more competition you face, the more important service becomes as a differentiator of your practice. Stanley Marcus, chairman emeritus of Neiman-Marcus specialty stores, sometimes says it this way: "The dollar bills the customer gets from the tellers in four banks are the same. What is different are the tellers." The Ritz Carlton hotel chain's philosophy is that employees build customer relationships, customer relationships build customer loyalty, and customer loyalty builds customer retention. You can't do it alone. You must have staff members who are kind, flexible, and responsive. Patients who have high expectations want staff to exhibit these traits. In order to maintain a staff to meet those expectations, you need to demonstrate leadership, use wise selection processes, provide training, and set an example.

Leadership

Football coach Paul "Bear" Bryant said, "If anything goes bad, I did it. If anything goes semi-good, we did it. If anything goes real good, you did it. That's all it takes to win football games" (Bryant and Underwood, 1974). Leaders respect the competence of every person in their organization. The single most critical factor in providing excellent service for patients is the culture you create. Be fanatical in your concern for patient safety and comfort so that it becomes the dominant theme in your organization. Every person on the team— physicians, other clinicians, and support staff alike—must share in demonstrating a caring attitude. Job descriptions, orientation programs, employee handbooks, and performance reviews should include patient satisfaction criteria. Without this information, how can staff members understand the direction you want the practice to take?

Do staff members understand how they contribute to the success of the practice? Are they interested in strengthening their relationships with others? Ask team members to complete the following sentences:

Referring physicians speak well of our practice when _____.

Patients are happy with our practice when _____.

Staff members are proud of our practice when _____.

Our practice is here to provide _____ to patients so that they see us as _____. We do this by _____.

If I could make one change to improve the quality of our practice, I would _____.

The problem patients encounter most frequently in our practice is _____.

Answers to these questions, such as those that follow, give operational meaning to your mission.

Referring physicians speak well of our practice when

Staff are responsive, knowledgeable, and accessible.

State-of-the-art equipment is available.

When the patient is returned to them.

When they know what is happening with their patient.

Patients are happy with our practice when

The expected clinical outcome is achieved.

Requests are responded to promptly and with kindness.

Staff are responsive, skilled, caring, and informed.

Patient education instructions are understandable.

Registration procedures are understandable and efficient.

Staff members are proud of our practice when

All staff are skilled, concerned, and caring.

All staff work together to increase quality.

Leadership communicates often.

Leadership recognizes employee contributions.

The practice has a good image.

New employees are proud to be part of the organization.

The answers your staff give will provide you with a sense of what they value most about your organization. If you take time to build consensus about those values, you will be helping employees know what action to take in all kinds of situations. Whatever your values are, they must be highly regarded, observed, and reinforced.

You can validate staff responses by asking patients and referring physicians the same questions. For example, you might ask patients to complete this sentence: "I am happy with the care I receive when _____." If your patients equate good care with being listened to and not receiving conflicting advice, you have additional information that helps you define what the practice should emphasize. Where staff and patient expectations are markedly different, you have identified an opportunity to develop strategies to create more realistic expectations.

People want to be part of something that has purpose. One primary care group developed a mission statement that emphasized that patients would always be seen, even when they arrived without an appointment. The practice leaders felt that their patient population was denied medical care because of financing, transportation, and other social problems. They did not want to be another barrier to care. The mission statement reminded everyone that fitting patients into the schedule was what the organization stood for. Effective mission statements define who the organization serves and the needs and expectations of those individuals.

Developing Your Staff's Image

Begin to define roles by how those roles benefit patients. Wouldn't you like to hear your receptionist describe his role as the person who helps patients feel welcome and less anxious when they arrive for appointments—instead of saying, "I'm just the receptionist"?

Do not refer to your female staff members as "girls." Would you call a girl if you had an important question to ask? Referring to adult women as girls doesn't inspire patients' confidence in them and makes you appear outdated.

If you don't have employees saying to you, "I love working here," you need to invest some time and energy in staff development. Every employee should feel like the employee of the month, every month. Think you're too busy to give that kind of attention to your staff? Then don't expect your staff to give world-class attention to your patients.

Excellent employees want the same quality of relationship with their employer that makes their other relationships succeed. Listening to your employees shows trust and respect, two vital qualities for successful relationships. An op-ed piece in the *Wall Street Journal* described the role of a consultant as one who charges $2,000 a day for advice that leaders could get from their employees for nothing. "Why do so many companies fail to capitalize on their employees' knowledge and expertise?" One reason: employees have too much to lose by telling leadership something it doesn't want to hear (Cantoni, 1997, p. A18).

Identifying Opportunities for Improvement

You want staff who are loyal to you, and loyalty includes letting you know when problems arise. Staff have to know that you want them to take responsibility. They may feel that you shouldn't be bothered because you're so busy. Tell staff that you're always going to be busy, that there will never be a good time, but that the earlier you learn of problems, the easier they are to resolve. What's more, you'd just as soon have the opportunity to figure out a solution before you're asked by patients to do so. FedEx uses the 1–10–100 concept developed by Organizational Dynamics Inc. to encourage early problem identification (*Blueprints for Service Quality*, 1994). The concept is that the cost of rectifying a problem increases with the length of time the company takes to fix it. If the problem is corrected immediately, it may cost $1. To fix it later might cost $10. If the problem reaches the customer, it might cost $100 to correct.

As a leader, one of your responsibilities should be to watch for sacred cows, those rules that have outlived their usefulness. One practice had an informal policy that only one employee and the service company could change the toner in the copier. Six months after the employee left the practice, patients were being inconvenienced whenever the toner needed replacement. It took a consultant to point out to leaders of the practice that the informal policy needed to be changed.

Develop solutions with, not for, staff. I once heard a story about a health club that equipped the showers with expensive shampoo. The shampoo bottles kept disappearing. Shortages would result, and clients were disappointed and sometimes angry. Management deliberated about what to do. Should they switch to cheaper shampoo that wouldn't be stolen? Should they raise membership fees to allow for shrinkage? Should they set up a system to check a shower after each use to make sure the bottles were still there? Unable to come up with a win-win solution, someone said, "Why don't we ask Joe? He's the locker room attendant, maybe he'll have an idea." Well, sure enough, he did. "No problem. I'll just take the caps off the shampoo bottles before I put them in the showers." When staff create solutions, they have a greater investment in making them succeed.

Encouraging Flexibility

Encourage staff members to be flexible with patients, because individual patient expectations vary. Give staff the freedom to customize service to individual needs.

How many rules do you have? Customer service guru Jan Carlzon (1996) told a story about a hotel that had been named in one survey as the number-one hotel in the world for ten consecutive years. Mr. Carlzon contacted the hotel to learn how it had accomplished this remarkable feat. The manager's reply was, "Well, I'm not exactly sure, but it may have something to do with our two rules." "What two rules?" asked Mr. Carlzon. Rule number one: an employee cannot say no to a customer. Rule number two: if an employee needs to say no, he or she must obtain the approval of a supervisor.

Do you make it easier for employees to say no than to say yes to patients? One way to find out is to examine every one of your rules and define how that rule benefits patients. For example, you may have a rule that a staff member must make a copy of the patient's insurance card at each visit. The benefit would be that when you have up-to-date information, the patient isn't bothered by unnecessary questions or claim denials by his insurance company. Defining the benefit of rules makes it easier for staff members to explain your rationale to patients. As part of this exercise, you can consider when exceptions will routinely need to be made to the rule.

Selecting and Orienting New Employees

If you think about any recent positive and negative experiences you have had with companies, at least one and probably both had to do with the attitude of an employee with whom you dealt. Working with staff members who are knowledgeable, enthusiastic, sincere, and friendly makes everyone's life a lot more pleasant. It's much easier to teach skills to a person with a positive attitude than it is to turn a negative attitude into a positive one. Flexibility, creativity, and a sense of humor are key attributes that enthusiastic people possess. As Ralph Waldo Emerson said, "Nothing great was ever accomplished without enthusiasm."

Where does genuinely caring behavior come from? Not from policies, equipment, locations, or networks. It comes from the people you hire and the training you give them. You'd like every staff member to have a strong work ethic and a compassionate heart.

Daniel Friend, CEO of Healthcare Solutions Group in Richmond, Virginia, asks applicants to describe the personalities of their previous patients and coworkers. The applicant's description says a great deal about his or her own personality. "If they say they were pleasant and cheerful, hire them. If they say they were demanding, impatient or otherwise not courteous, then the applicant is not personable." Friend also asks his receptionist to evaluate applicants as they arrive and wait for the interview to begin (Daniel Friend, personal communication with the author, 1997).

When interviewing applicants, ask them about what they would do in various practice situations: "What would you do if . . . ?" Observe the applicants' attitude about the scenarios they describe. Do they take ownership of situations requiring their assistance? How do they feel about what they do? Also ask applicants to tell you about a time when they had to give bad news to their boss.

The time to make sure that your values are consistent with those of your new employee is before that employee ever begins working for you. Knowing what your values are and how they are practiced in your organization is critical in determining compatibility. For example, the practice that never turns patients away could ask prospective employees how they reacted when their schedule became hectic because of drop-in patients. Or how flexible they could be about lunch breaks.

Being able to describe the important aspects of your mission helps job applicants determine whether their skills and personalities match the needs of your practice. One practice defined its mission as follows: "Our primary concern is for the comfort of our patients. In the short term, we accomplish this by helping them feel welcome and comfortable during each visit. In the long term, we accomplish this by encouraging them in compliance and healthy living habits." The team members identified actions that would support these values, such as greeting patients by name, respecting patient confidentiality, and keeping patients informed about what to expect. They also looked for job candidates who had experience with or a passion for patient education and behavior modification. At Southwest Airlines, loyal customers are invited to help select flight attendants for employment with the airline, which is another way of determining if prospective employees will succeed in Southwest's customer service–oriented environment.

There is no better time to educate staff on what you expect than at orientation. In his book *Empires of the Mind*, Denis Waitley (1995, p. 73) tells the story of a nurse on her first day of work in a surgical unit. At the end of a procedure, she informed the surgeon that the sponge count was off, that only eleven of the twelve sponges were accounted for. The surgeon told her that he had removed them all and was ready to close. She objected. He told her he would take responsibility. The nurse protested again: "Think of the patient!" The surgeon then uncovered the sponge under his foot and said with a smile, "You'll do just fine in this or any other hospital."

Without an orientation program, people may do things the way they have always done them, and there are usually positives and negatives associated with this. During orientation at a managed care company, a new employee mentioned that she had found she could get rid of complaining customers quickly by suggesting that they would get quicker action by calling OSHA to report their problem. Considering that she had been hired to work in provider relations, this was not the response her new employer wanted. Without the orientation program, they might never have discovered her preferred manner of handling patient complaints about professionals participating in the network.

Make employees feel valued from the first day. Physicians should take time to greet new employees and tell them personally how important they are to the success of the practice and how important it is to identify and manage patient expectations.

Training

Are you investing as much in staff as you are in equipment and technology? In one study of good and bad surprises as reported by hospital patients (Nelson and Larson, 1993), no one mentioned the appearance of hospital facilities. Instead, participants commented on the interpersonal aspects of care, the amount of attention they received, perks, and how their family and friends were treated. If staff members are to feel comfortable in their roles, you must provide education and training regarding the quality of interactions with patients. If your staff members don't know what you expect, how will they know what to do? Do they have enough information to act in the ways you want them to act? Without direction, staff members will be inconsistent in their attention to patient concerns. Another benefit of training is that it's better to fail in the classroom than with the patient.

The good news is that there are countless opportunities for training. Magazines, newspapers, television shows, and movies all provide customer service material on a regular basis. Just reading the newspaper can provide you with food for thought and discussion. The *New York Times* published this letter from reader Alan Loflin (Alexander, 1997, p. C2).

> I was in Penn Station purchasing Amtrak tickets to Wilmington, Del. when a woman approached the agent at the next window.
>
> "Is it your job to sell me a ticket to anywhere I want to go?" she asked.
>
> "Yes, ma'am," he replied. "Where would you like to go?"
>
> "To hell and back," she answered.
>
> Without batting an eye, the agent, with utmost courtesy, consulted his computer screen and said "Sorry, ma'am, but that train is completely sold out."

One of the goals of training is to eliminate obstacles. People create obstacles when they say the wrong things to patients, either thoughtlessly or because of bad habits. For example, there are two ways to say almost anything. A few years ago, the New York City Taxicab Commission developed suggested responses for cab drivers to use when answering customer complaints. Printed on clipboards, the responses were helpful to drivers who might otherwise have said the first (rude) thing that occurred to them. Some health care examples are shown in Exhibit 9.1.

Training programs that can help staff members manage patient expectations include programs on informed consent, effective listening, interviewing, participatory decision making, handling complaints, anticipating and resolving problems, and counseling. In addition, when you make it possible for your staff to visit physicians and organizations that you refer to, staff members gain firsthand knowledge that will help them manage patient expectations.

Exhibit 9.1. Eliminating Obstacles.

Instead of saying . . .	Consider . . .
"We don't handle that here."	"At this office, we handle . . . What I can do is give you the telephone number of the office that can help you."
"I don't know where she is."	"She's unavailable at the moment."
"It's crazy here today."	"It seems that many of our patients need us today."
"You're wrong."	"Let me see if I can clarify this situation."
"What is this regarding?"	"May I leave a message with your name and telephone number? Is there any other information that would be helpful for Dr._____ to have before she returns your call?"
"Are you a new patient?"	"When did you last visit us?"
"I'll have to check on that."	"I'll be happy to check on that."
"I'm just the receptionist."	"Paul is the best person to answer that question for you. May I put you on hold while I see if he's available?"
"I can't."	"I won't be able to because . . ."
"I'll be honest with you . . ." or, "To tell you the truth . . ."	Saying what you mean to say. Don't you always tell the truth?
"I don't know."	"May I check on that for you and call you back?"
"We can see you today, but you'll have to be here by 3:00 P.M."	"Yes, we can see you today. Can you be sure to be here by 3:00 P.M.?"
"No."	Paraphrasing. Tell what you can do and why. For example: "Mr. Mallozzi, I understand that you would like us to refill your prescription. Dr. D'Angelo needs to see you to personally ensure that you receive the most appropriate medication. I can make an appointment for you this afternoon."
"Oh boy, did we mess up."	"I'm sorry this occurred. To correct this situation for you, I am going to . . . Thank you for bringing it to my attention, and please call me again if you need me in the future."
"Next?"	"How may I help you?"
"You'll have to . . ."	"Here's how we handle that. Please _____."

Lifetime Value of a Patient

Most patients are happier with long-term relationships. They feel comfortable knowing how to access and work through systems. They don't want to explain their special circumstances over and over again.

Taking a serious look at the lifetime value of a patient is a real eye opener about the value of long-term relationships. The lifetime value of a customer is a concept with which all members of the organization should be familiar. It only makes sense that an item worth $73,000 will be handled more carefully than an item worth $73. The patient who comes in for a blood test is not a $73 patient. He can't be replaced with another $73 patient. He is instead the annual revenue generated by caring for him multiplied by the number of years he could be expected to remain with the practice, plus the revenues of the other patients he could have referred to you for care.

Patient retention is vital to the success of your organization, and it should receive greater attention from you than attracting new patients. The impact of losing any patient is immediate. Experts say that it costs five times as much to replace a lost customer as it does to retain an existing one. Associated with the new patient are the additional costs of setting up a medical record, updating the computer system, orienting the patient to the practice, and so on. Employees should understand that they are responsible not merely for managing a transaction but for cementing a relationship. And it may not be just the relationship with one patient that is affected. These days, a lost patient can mean a lost contract with a managed care company or employer.

Staff Meetings

How do you begin each day with your team? Do you greet them warmly? Do you ask about their families or something else that is going on in their lives? Are you upbeat about the day ahead? Even a five-minute pep talk in the morning to review the list of patients being seen during the day can make a huge difference. Some practices begin each day by giving a cheer: "Who are we here for? Our patients!" Sounds corny, but it sets the tone for the day. A brief morning meeting gives everyone the opportunity to be aware of which patients require extra time and attention, who will be having procedures or testing, and so on. Errors are often made when someone knows something but fails to tell someone else. Faulty communication among physicians and staff makes patients nervous. In addition to quick morning briefings, regularly scheduled staff meetings help prevent mistakes.

Work with your staff to develop the ground rules for staff meetings. They may make such suggestions as the following:

- Have full participation.

- Start and end on time.

- Conduct one conversation at a time.

- Arrive at closure on issues.

- Have an agenda before each meeting.

- Clarify and understand responsibilities and actions.

- Bring up and discuss troubling issues quickly. If someone thinks there will be a problem, there will be a problem.

- Have fun.

- Schedule the next meeting at the end of each meeting.

Some practices begin their meetings with staff sharing stories about exceptional patient service they have provided or observed. Or you might ask staff members to recall early memories of visiting a physician and then talk about what actions created lasting impressions. Urge individuals to thank other members of the team for any assistance provided since the last meeting. Also encourage staff members to attend networking meetings and then report at staff meetings on what they have learned.

Staff feedback is as important as patient feedback in improving the quality of care and service provided by your practice. Don't have a thirty-minute staff meeting and monopolize twenty-five minutes of it. Use staff meetings to create an atmosphere in which staff will suggest improvements based on what they hear from patients; reward ideas; talk about ways to strengthen relationships with patients and with their own business and personal contacts as sources of referrals.

How many suggestions do you receive and implement per employee per year? How well do you execute those ideas?

Dealing with Change

Effective leaders understand that change creates anxiety and that a natural response is to feel that the traditional way of doing things is the correct way or that exception can be taken to suggestions for change. But as author Tom Hopkins (1982, p. 79) says, "The pain of every change is forgotten when the benefits of that change are realized." Articulate the need for change in a way that benefits employees. Ask them to develop annual objectives that focus on learning new skills. Employees could be asked to complete their objectives in this format: "Learn _____ so that I can _____." This strategy helps staff members develop the habit of anticipating and adapting to change. Employees start to feel more confident about their ability to cope with even unwanted change.

Help staff members get what they want. If you listen, your employees will tell you what matters to them. For some, it's the respect of their family. For others, it might be to advance in their profession. Think creatively about how you can contribute to the successful accomplishment of each employee's goals. For one employee, job security was of paramount importance. The practice manager was able to show him how cross-training would make him more

valuable to the organization and protect him in the event of down-
sizing. The practice manager also pointed out that additional skills
would enable the employee to find other employment easily if the
need arose. The employee was only too happy to take on extra responsibility in pursuit of his personal goal.

Your own ability to reframe situations, to find opportunities in
problems, sends a clear message to your staff about the resiliency of
your organization. Think before you react in front of staff members
when you receive information about changes that you haven't anticipated, such as new regulations from the government or a managed care company.

Setting an Example

All the training in the world won't achieve what you want unless
you are also setting a good example. Your credibility depends on the
example you set. Without example, staff members will listen to your
latest management philosophy and think to themselves, "This too
shall pass."

Albert Schweitzer said, "Example is not the main thing in influencing others. It is the only thing." Some experts believe that
companies don't need a mission or values statement if they have
leaders who lead by example. Steven Berglas (1997, p. 33), a psychologist on the faculty at Harvard Medical School, says, "You want
to know how leadership works? Throw out the mission statements;
don't bother with values statements; just look at how the organization's leader behaves and you'll know with 100 percent certainty
how employees will behave."

One of my favorite stories is about Mahatma Gandhi. He was
visited one day by a woman and her young son, and the woman
asked, "Gandhi, please tell my son to stop eating sugar."

"Please return in two weeks," replied Gandhi. The woman went
away and returned with the child two weeks later. "Gandhi, please
tell my son to stop eating sugar," she requested again.

This time, Gandhi looked at the little boy and said, "Stop eating sugar."

Confused, the woman asked Gandhi, "Why didn't you tell him that two weeks ago?"

Gandhi replied, "Because two weeks ago, I was eating sugar" (Millman, 1980, p. 185).

Can you still perform the functions you require entry-level personnel to perform? Are leaders required to attend all training sessions provided for frontline staff? Leadership has always been more about passion than administration. You express your passion for providing excellent patient care and service through the example you set.

People want to follow optimistic leaders. Smile and let others see that you enjoy what you do. Ronald Reagan changed American sentiment through the way he enjoyed the presidency. How bad could things be, people thought, if the president, with all his responsibilities, was having such a good time? Instead of looking decades older at the end of his terms, as many of his predecessors had, Reagan looked as good leaving office as he did entering it. Do you look as good at the end of the day or week as you do at the beginning? People are drawn to people who love what they do. Start smiling. You'll feel a difference in yourself and in the responsiveness of others.

If you expect your staff to be unfailingly courteous and compassionate, you have to consistently exhibit those same qualities. In his book *The Seven Habits of Highly Effective People,* Stephen Covey (1989, p. 58) writes, "Always treat your employees exactly as you want them to treat your best customer." What does it say if you tell your staff to address all patients by name but you don't know all of your employees' names? You shouldn't roll your eyes to the ceiling when you're speaking about a difficult patient unless you want your staff to do the same thing. Always speak well of your staff. When my mother was engaged to be married, a friend gave her some valuable advice: "Don't ever speak ill of your husband to another. Later,

you'll forget what you said, but the other person will remember." At
a hospital medical staff gathering, one physician talked about his
"BMW" team—a staff he described as "bitchers, moaners, and whin-
ers." Do you wonder why he had a problem with high turnover?

Although some people seem to enjoy it, negativity does nothing to enhance your career or your life. Negativity is contagious and
affects both patient and staff interactions, damaging the overall performance of your practice. If someone in your practice is hopelessly
negative, free up his future so that he can try to be happy elsewhere.
Sometimes, people fall into a pattern of negativity without realizing it. Create a paper or mental chart for yourself. Check to see how
many negative statements and how many positive statements you
make in the next hour. Ask yourself: How would you like to have
you for a boss, physician, spouse, friend? Why, and why not? Then,
start doing more of the positives and fewer of the negatives.

Recognizing Staff Members

Employees need to know that their abilities and loyalties are appreciated. When was the last time you recognized a staff member?
Never? Are you quick to criticize when people do a poor job but
prone to take them for granted when things go smoothly? It's critically important to acknowledge the contributions of your staff. Bob
Hope was once asked why he didn't retire and go fishing. "Because
fish don't applaud," he replied (Harmetz, 1989, p. C1). Positive reinforcement is the key to changing an existing behavior, teaching
a new one, or enhancing the positive attitudes and behaviors that
already exist. A sincere compliment costs nothing, takes little time,
and is often long remembered by the recipient. Don't let opportunities for recognition slip by.

Ritz Carlton hotels have cards printed with "First Class!" at the
top and "Ritz Carlton" and its logo at the bottom, with space for a
handwritten note. The cards are readily available for employee-to-
employee recognition (Schneiderman, 1996). At Kendle, a company

that performs clinical trials for pharmaceuticals, employee photographs line the walls. The black-and-white photos show each employee with symbols of his or her nonwork interests, from
grandchildren to scuba diving equipment.

The larger your organization is, the harder it is for senior leadership to spot opportunities for recognition. Goldsmith (1996) cites
one example of how to deal with this difficulty: the CEO of a
telecommunications company asks his division-level executives to
send him a quarterly report regarding exceptional employees. The
CEO calls each one to recognize his or her contribution and to ask
how the company can increase its effectiveness.

If you begin using positive reinforcement tomorrow, you'll begin
seeing results tomorrow. In the words of Goethe, "If you treat men
the way they are, you never improve them. If you treat them the
way you want them to be, you do."

◆   ◆   ◆   ◆   ◆   ◆   ◆

The author Elbert Hubbard said, "Be pleasant until ten o'clock in
the morning and the rest of the day will take care of itself." Patients
see and feel your organization's atmosphere, so be sure that positive
statements to your staff and staff recognition are part of your every-
day routine.

10

Informed Consent

Life is short, the art long, opportunity fleeting,
experiment treacherous, judgment difficult.

Hippocrates

One of the best opportunities you have to bring expectations and anticipated outcomes into alignment is the consent discussion. By considering patient expectations along with the patient's general medical condition, the duration and severity of his symptoms, the anticipated outcome, and the risk factors, you help the patient decide whether the projected outcome will meet his needs.

The consent process should begin early in the relationship. Rather than being merely a recitation of risks, benefits, and alternatives, consent should be an interactive exchange of relevant information designed to mutually explore expectations and understanding of pertinent clinical issues (Holzer, 1991).

Consent has been likened to the sales process—persuading the patient to accept what medicine has to offer. But it should be much more participatory than that. One of the alternatives in every consent discussion should be that the patient can choose to do nothing. The patient then clearly understands that he is in control of the choices he will make—it is an appropriate place to start, considering the current era, in which patients have both a "buyer beware" attitude and access to tremendous amounts of medical information.

Advise patients about the nature of the proposed treatment and the risks, benefits, and alternatives, including the alternative of doing nothing. Then ask, "What questions can I answer for you?" The patient may not verbalize his questions but is likely to be asking himself, "Why is this a good idea? Is it worth the risk, cost, and time?"

After discussing the treatment and answering questions, ask your patient, "Now that we have discussed the nature of the procedure and the risks, benefits, and alternatives, including the alternative of doing nothing, what would you like me to do?" The patient who can't answer that question or who says, "Whatever you think best," is not adequately prepared to give informed consent. Patients frequently ask the physician what her choice would be. When you reflect on what you would recommend for yourself or a family member, be as honest as possible while also keeping your patient's circumstances and expectations in mind.

The benefit of pursuing consent in this way is that when a patient participates in the decision, there is more confidence about moving forward. Providing complete information about a diagnosis decreases uncertainty and anxiety (Stull, Lo, and Charles, 1984). In addition, the patient who accepts responsibility for the decision may be less likely to sue if things do not turn out the way you or he had anticipated.

If the format of your consent discussions is different from what most patients expect, be sure to explain your rationale to patients ahead of time. One day, a patient was waiting in the reception area to meet with his physician prior to having a vasectomy. Another patient was called by the nurse first. The first patient was called next and was surprised to find himself in the physician's office with the other patient. The physician conducted the consent discussion with both men simultaneously. Perhaps it comes as no surprise that neither man asked any questions during the meeting.

Helping Patients Choose

Take time to understand *how* your patient makes choices. Some people prefer to delegate decisions to others; some want help only when they feel they need it; some want all available information before making a decision; and still others seek no information beyond what you tell them. Is your patient the type who subscribes to *Consumer Reports* and reviews it carefully before making a purchase? Is he the type who will buy whatever his spouse wants?

Help patients make informed decisions by helping them anticipate how they will feel after the procedure. Whereas some will think of the long-term benefit, others will give greater weight to how they will feel in the near term. Ask patients about the aspect of the illness they would most like to avoid.

Asking patients about their understanding of the procedure is an important means of identifying expectations:

> DOCTOR: Have you known anyone who has had this operation? What was his experience like?
>
> PATIENT: It was wonderful. I saw him riding his bike two days later.
>
> DOCTOR: Ah, two days later. Well, that's pretty unusual. Most patients don't feel up to physical exercise for at least a week.

> **Ask patients about the aspect of the illness they would most like to avoid.**

Paraphrasing what the patient tells you gives you an opportunity to correct any misconceptions or misstatements. In this example, the patient might reply, "Oh, Doctor, did I say two days later? I meant two weeks later."

Patients who participate in decision making regarding their care have better follow-through and better outcomes. A patient's values and beliefs will often have a significant impact on his willingness to proceed with a proposed treatment plan. Increased patient participation in decision making can take place only if you pay attention to patients' beliefs and perceptions, particularly if these are distorted in any way (Buchanan and others, 1996). During your meeting to talk about consent, remember that the discussion is about the person as much as about the condition being considered. Making a note in the chart regarding the patient's rationale reflects a serious consent discussion and can remind you of this factor in the future.

Patient satisfaction is so highly correlated with a physician's participatory style that many satisfaction surveys ask patients to report how much they participated in decision making about their treatment. In one study (Kaplan and others, 1995), physicians were ranked according to how participatory their style was. Physicians who ranked in the highest quartile for participatory style had far fewer patients leaving their practices than did those in the lowest quartile.

Agreeing to the treatment and following through with it are two very different things. Following through with the treatment plan is an intermediate outcome measure that presumes the expected health outcome will follow. The patient's initiative in adhering to the agreed-upon treatment plan significantly affects the eventual outcome. Organizations accepting risk must have strategies in place to influence outcomes. However, when the treatment plan interferes with the patient's lifestyle or the achievement of other goals, failure to follow through is a real possibility. The patient's belief about the benefit of the treatment is often a determining factor in whether he will comply. Patient follow-through is addressed in Chapter Fourteen.

Using the Consent Process to Manage Patient Expectations

Physicians sometimes say to me, "If I tell the patient all the things that can go wrong, he won't have the operation." Simply stated, if the patient is a competent adult, it's his choice, not yours.

Advise patients that complications do occur. Some physicians fear that telling patients that mistakes are possible will lead to increased anxiety and to lack of trust in the physician. In an interview on teaching residents and medical students to disclose mistakes, Albert Wu of Johns Hopkins said, "While you don't want patients to completely lose faith in the medical profession, the more they realize that physicians are human beings and the more they participate in decision making and share responsibility for things that happen, the more realistic their expectations are" (Keyes and Augello, 1997, p. 6). Steve Stelovich (1997) of Harvard Pilgrim Health Care, Massachusetts, believes that anticipating the likelihood of patients having a bad outcome after a specific procedure enables a physician to remember to discuss possibilities and consequences with patients. "Anticipating in this sense would be more than reciting the risks and benefits of a procedure. It might involve discussing the patient's likely post-surgical symptoms with the patient's family and explaining which of these are not worrisome as well as which symptoms warrant follow-up" (p. 8). Stelovich also emphasizes educating patients and families about their role in preventing errors.

Harold J. Bursztajn (1997), a forensic psychiatrist and author of *Medical Choices, Medical Chances: How Patients, Families and Physicians Can Cope with Uncertainty*, has said that "lawsuits typically are triggered neither by actual medical negligence nor by tragic outcomes alone, but rather by tragic outcomes combined with bad feelings and alienated relationships. Strong treatment alliances prevent patients from filing lawsuits. In such an alliance, informed consent is not a mere signature on a checklist of risks, but a process of mutual engagement with clinical realities and the feelings that accompany them." Bursztajn warns that taping of the consent discussion can create adversarial situations.

Patients who are told what to expect are in a better position to prepare and adapt. Thus the consent discussion should always include a timetable of what can be expected to happen next.

Preventing Malpractice Through the Sharing of Uncertainty

Patients don't always appreciate that there are risks and side effects associated with medicine. Patients want to place their faith in technology and medications. It's an adjustment for many patients to find out that there isn't a pill for everything and that their expectations are unrealistic. Gutheil, Bursztajn, and Brodsky (1984) point out that patients who present with unrealistic expectations need empathy. They advise physicians to empathize with the patient's unrealistic wishes and then modify the patient's expectations. For example, the physician might say, "I wish I could give you a medication that was sure to have only positive side effects."

Some physicians hope to cover all the bases by saying that anything is possible, that the patient could die as a result of the procedure—no matter how minor that procedure might be. It is not enough to tell patients to expect the unexpected. They have a right to know and you have a duty to inform them of the most likely things that will take place. Telling a patient that anything can happen, even death, when death is a remote possibility, may lead him to discount all your admonitions about potential complications.

A Scottish study of surgical patients (Finlay, Atkinson, and Moos, 1995) found that patients with unrealistic expectations were more likely to express dissatisfaction with their outcomes in the early postoperative stages. To help make patients expectations more realistic, the researchers recommended adequate patient preparation prior to surgery, supplemented by the use of printed literature.

There is a difference, however, between positive expectations and unrealistic expectations. Positive expectations should not be dampened. Researchers at the University of California, Los Angeles, found that positive expectations were generally associated with good mood, adjustment to illness, and quality of life, even in patients who experienced health setbacks (Leedham, Meyerowitz, Muirhead, and Frist, 1995). High preoperative expectations predicted later adherence to a complex medical regimen. Patients' self-reported positive expectations have been found to be generally associated with adjustment to the illness and adherence to a complex medical regimen.

Using Tools That Support the Consent Process

Consent forms have several advantages. You can use a consent form to help guide your discussion, provide detailed information, and save time in documentation. Watch out for forms that are too technical for a layperson to understand, and be sure to update your consent forms regularly.

Consent forms can be an effective means of assuring yourself that the patient understands what he is agreeing to. However, forms cannot substitute for the consent discussion. Forms have given some physicians a (false) sense of security that as long as the patient signs a form, there is proof that the patient gave his informed consent. These physicians often ask staff members to obtain the patient's signature on the consent form when no discussion with the patient has taken place. The most blatant example is that of a patient being asked to sign a form that begins with the words, "Dr. Smith has discussed with me . . . ," when in fact the patient has never even met Dr. Smith. Whereas obtaining a patient's *signature* on a consent form can be delegated, obtaining the patient's *consent*—the consent discussion itself—must always be done by the physician.

Consent forms can be helpful in providing information, but they have less educational benefit for the patient when you do not provide him with a copy. In one hospital, a patient was asked to sign a consent form for a minor surgical procedure. He read the form, signed it, then asked for a copy. Two levels of managers had to be consulted before his request could be granted.

When patients are shown, rather than just told, about their problems, they have a better learning experience. For some, seeing is believing. Tim Shea of Concord, California, developed a consent kit for his patients contemplating foot surgery. The kit contains a description of the procedure, a copy of the consent form the patient will be asked to sign, a Betadine scrub (to indicate that it is a surgical procedure), and an application for the State of California Temporary Disabled Parking Permit. When Dr. Shea has the consent discussion with patients, they say, "Well, I won't need this permit, I'm not going to be disabled."

"You're not going be sick, as in stuck in bed," he replies, "but you are going to be disabled for a time." Shea is clear about what signs and symptoms should be reported to him right away. After surgery, when patients realize that foot surgery can be painful, they recall the conversation and are not upset that they are in more pain than they expected (Tim Shea, letter to the author, 1998).

Avoid the situation in which you explain the treatment for a child to one parent and find later that the other parent, whom you may not even have met, has signed the consent form.

•   •   •   •   •   •   •

Patients come to expect a certain outcome, based on any combination of the factors discussed in Part One of this book. If that outcome is not achieved, they may find fault with the physician. Take advantage of the consent discussion to see that your patients' expectations are realistic.

11

Patient Education

*It's not what you say that counts. It's what they hear
and absorb that really matters.*

Red Auerbach

E ffective patient education is giving personalized information just
in advance of or concurrent with a patient's need for it. Effective patient education gives patients the information and skills to
assume their own responsibility for care.

Helping Patients Be Right

In his book *Keeping the Edge: Giving Customers the Service They Demand,* Dick Schaaf (1995, p. 109) wrote: "In Japan, one school of
thought holds that the purpose of marketing is nothing less than
customer education: teaching the customer how to be right and
when to be satisfied."

The American Society of Internal Medicine publishes a brochure
titled "Communication—It's Good for Your Health" to help patients
know what information they should gather before a medical visit.
For example, readers are advised that their current problem, symptoms, medical history, family medical history, current medications,
personal habits, life changes, and allergies will all be important

factors in treatment, diagnosis, and outcomes. The brochure also addresses what patients should learn during a medical visit and the importance of compliance and follow-up. Patients are also advised to let their physician know about their expectations: "Have you told your doctor the kind of information you want?" the brochure asks.

Don't neglect giving information because of assumptions. Avoid medical jargon. Yes, your patients watch medical dramas on television, but they don't watch them with a medical dictionary in their hands. Avoid medical jargon even with health professionals. One nurse who had worked for many years in adult medicine told a story about joining a pediatric practice. On her first day of employment, lab results were phoned in, and she gave them to the physician. "Who are these results for?" the physician asked. The nurse answered, "Oh, I wrote it on the slip. They are for Billy Rubin."

When a diagnosis is a complete surprise to the patient, you will need to give the patient more information. A schoolteacher told me of her diagnosis of lupus. She knew nothing about lupus and had never known anyone who had been diagnosed with it. Her physician referred to her condition not as lupus but as a disease of her immune system. She interpreted this as AIDS and went home to a sleepless night of questioning how she might have contracted the disease. When she telephoned her physician the next day to ask him about it, he defined her condition as lupus and apologized for confusing her. The relationship with her physician continued successfully thanks to his handling of the misunderstanding. He didn't scoff at her or try to discredit what she remembered by saying something like, "You must not have been listening. I did say it was lupus." Instead, he empathized with her and offered to give her some written information about her condition. When patients have no prior experience with a procedure or condition, more comprehensive education may reduce the discrepancy between expectations and eventual outcomes.

Help your patients do the correct thing. When I take a train to New York City, I purchase a peak and an off-peak ticket for the round trip. My favorite ticket agent bends the off-peak ticket and reminds me that the folded ticket is for the afternoon trip. He spares me the possible embarrassment of trying to use a discounted ticket at the wrong time. Written information can also increase a patient's chances of being right. Many drivers leaving the parking garage at Children's Hospital in Boston ask the attendant for directions. The attendant gives the driver a four-by-six-inch card with directions to all the major routes. The written information is unexpected and especially appreciated by parents who have crying children with them.

Written information for even the simplest things means increased patient follow-through and satisfaction, and fewer telephone calls for you later. Written information reinforces what you have said and is particularly important when you are advising a person about more than one thing. For patients at risk for complications, written information is vital, because they are left to watch for those complications themselves. What should the patient expect? When should he call you?

People have a need to be right. Preventing litigation requires that you avoid discounting what patients tell you. When patients or their family members express a perception or opinion and the physician summarily rejects it, they feel insulted. If their opinions subsequently turn out to be correct, they may become angry and seek revenge. A malpractice suit is a means of forcing a physician to share the anger and distress that the patient is experiencing. In a study of plaintiff depositions (Beckman, Markakis, Suchman, and Frankel, 1994), researchers found that a sense of feeling discounted pervaded the depositions of patients suing for malpractice.

When a patient expects something that you can't give, find out why he wants it. The patient may be demanding a medication because a friend's health improved after taking it. Explain that the same disease can affect different individuals differently, and then review the patient's medical problems and treatment choices in a thoughtful manner.

When you are instructing a patient on how to self-administer a test or treatment, take time to watch him be successful. It's the best way to help your patient feel confident that he is performing successfully. This is a valuable opportunity to correct techniques or misunderstandings immediately, not at a later follow-up visit.

Access to Patient Education

Providing health information is one way to convey your interest in your patient's well-being. One practice has worked out an arrangement with a local bookstore. The bookstore provides copies of health-related books for the reception area. The physicians and staff write short reviews of the books on index cards and place them in the books. A sign advises patients that the books will be sent to them with no postage or handling charge by simply telephoning the bookstore with the name of the book and a credit card number for payment. This win-win-win situation benefited the patients, the practice, and the bookstore.

Take advantage of the health information services available from your system, network, hospital, managed care companies, and community agencies. Their information and services are often available at no charge for your patients. If a patient is helped by a program, take a moment to send a thank-you note to the program sponsor. It will be appreciated and may generate future referrals for you.

In a study of fifty women who received patient education materials at a multidisciplinary breast clinic (Vetto, Dubois, and Vetto, 1996), researchers found that only twenty-nine of the fifty remembered receiving the information, but of the twenty-nine, twenty-seven read the information, and half of those shared the materials with other women. Because patients may share your educational information with friends, it's a good idea to include your name and telephone number on that information. I was with a group of doctors at the Sheraton Palace Hotel in San Francisco. After meeting all day, we went out to a restaurant for dinner. While there, two of the doctors realized that they had left laptop computers in the conference room. Could I call the hotel and check to see if they were still there? Well, who knows the telephone number of a hotel they are visiting? The Sheraton Palace has its telephone number printed on the room keys. By recognizing a potential or actual customer need, the hotel helped us solve a problem quickly. Having your name and telephone number on everything you give or send to patients can reduce their anxiety in similar circumstances—when they need to call you from out of town, for example.

Audiocassettes of discharge instructions can be an effective substitute for printed information, particularly for patients with vision impairments. Patients can listen to the tape for clarification or reinforcement, and they can invite their family members to listen as well.

Technology is creating ever-changing definitions of how service should be delivered. When Medline became free for Internet users, the site immediately began receiving one million visits per day. When our twelve-year-old son tore the ACL ligament in his knee, I began telephoning colleagues to obtain recommendations for physicians and treatment options. My husband turned to the Internet. Within minutes, he had in his hands the definitive article comparing treatment outcomes for children under the age of fourteen with ACL injuries.

Because of rapid changes in medical information, you may not want to purchase large quantities of patient education materials. Many associations, including the American Academy of Child and Adolescent Psychiatry and the American Academy of Family Physicians, provide patient education sheets via the Internet. Both organizations give permission to duplicate the information for patients.

Focus-group and membership surveys told Kaiser that its members wanted better access to the company, closer relationships with their physicians, and access to good health information. A pilot group of Kaiser members have access to a Web site that allows them to schedule nonurgent appointments, search for disease-specific information, participate in discussion groups, and send questions to nurses, pharmacists, and other specialists. Enhancements being considered include ordering prescription refills and sending e-mail directly to physicians.

Interactive technology can be used to provide understandable yet comprehensive information to help patients consider treatment options. Some shared decision making programs allow patients to make decisions in their own homes, at their own pace.

Clinical Guidelines

Some physicians order tests and medications because a patient expects them to. Although interpersonal skills could be used to modify those patient expectations, time constraints may prevent physicians from using those skills.

Clinical guidelines are a patient education tool that can be quite effective in managing patient expectations. *Business & Health* reported that three-quarters of physician respondents to a Reed Group survey said that they are asked about twice each week to extend the amount of time patients can take off from work ("Doc, Can't You Give Me . . . ," 1995). Half of the physicians found that sharing written guidelines specifying the number of days allowed for a particular illness or injury helped change patient expectations. Clinical guidelines can serve as prompts to remind physicians that certain tests or follow-ups are needed. They can also help physicians be more consistent in treatment and may serve as protection from unrealistic expectations and frivolous malpractice claims.

Another study (Shulkin and Ferniany, 1996) looked at whether sharing critical pathways with cardiac bypass graft surgery patients would lead to realistic expectations that would in turn lead to higher patient satisfaction. The researchers recommended that sharing a critical pathway might have a greater effect if the path was shared with the patient before admission, while he was being seen in his physician's office. They also suggested that developing a video version of the critical pathway be considered.

Numerous sources now provide guidelines written specifically for patients to help them decide on appropriate care. Some of these guidelines have incorporated patient preferences. Guidelines may help patients decide not to seek care when self-treatment is an option or when a condition is probably self-limiting. In addition to saving money, guidelines may improve patients' health status, boost follow-through, and prevent costly complications by encouraging early treatment when warranted. Stay informed about the availability of guidelines. An excellent resource to assist you in staying current might be the quality improvement manager or health sciences librarian at your hospital.

When you change practice patterns as a result of new or revised clinical guidelines, share the information with patients. If a patient has always been given an appointment with the physician for a certain symptom but is suddenly being seen by a physician assistant or nurse practitioner, he should know why the change has occurred. In addition, be sure that your patient education materials reflect the guidelines you decide to follow.

Support Groups

Patients are often adamant that the only people who can understand them are others who are experiencing or have experienced the same suffering. One orthopedic surgeon arranges for patients to speak with former patients who have undergone the surgery being considered. He tries to match patients by age and interest. After surgery, patients have the opportunity to help future patients in the same way.

Support groups can help patients manage emotional reactions to pain, cope with their condition, and resume their activities of

daily living. Support groups can be an effective way for you to provide additional patient education without a corresponding investment of your time.

•   •   •   •   •   •   •

Education inspires confidence, helps patients reach their personal
objectives, and prevents unpleasant surprises. Take advantage of
teachable moments, those times when the patient is asking questions, when the patient is pain free and comfortable, or when the
patient identifies problems. You will simultaneously help manage
your patient's expectations and increase your credibility with the
patient.

12

Best Practices

> *Keep on the lookout for novel and interesting ideas*
> *that others have used successfully. Your idea has to be*
> *original only in its adaptation to the problem you're*
> *currently working on.*
>
> Thomas Edison

Determining best practices is the process of finding out who does something best, examining how they do it, and considering whether their strategies are transferable to your practice. Finding innovative ways to adapt the successes of companies outside of health care can create a competitive advantage for your practice. This chapter addresses several best practice strategies that can help you identify and respond to your patients' expectations.

Assume the Patient's Role

A Press Ganey survey of one million hospital patients released in January 1997 revealed that staff sensitivity to the inconvenience of illness and hospitalization was a key driver of patient satisfaction ("Empathy Beats Fancy Food . . . ," 1997). Staff can heighten their sensitivity by listening to patients and imagining what it is like to be in their situations.

Some of a physician's greatest insights result from her experiences as a patient. The Irish have a saying, "The wearer best knows where the shoe pinches." Experiencing the company as a customer is a best practice technique used by many successful companies. Banks ask employees to complete deposit slips while three of their fingers are taped together to simulate the experience of a customer with arthritis. Restaurants ask employees to read menus while wearing glasses covered with translucent film to simulate the experience of a customer with impaired vision. A computer executive brought his management team to the loading dock and gave each manager a computer to assemble, using the company's instruction manual as the only guide. British Airways customer service representatives fly with customers to experience service firsthand from the customer's perspective.

Many companies give their employees product samples to use. This helps staff be optimally knowledgeable about those products when customers have questions. Their testing of the product, combined with comprehensive product training, enables them to honestly discuss whether and how the product will meet the customer's needs. Their individual experience using a product will not be identical to the customer's but will assist them in managing customer expectations.

Some hospital residency programs encourage residents to pose as patients undergoing tests. After the experience, residents are more likely to knock before entering patient rooms and to explain to patients why procedures and tests are needed and when the results of tests will be available (Turner, 1995).

Becoming a patient is a transformational experience for many people. Roles often change when illness occurs. When physicians and staff undergo that transformation, they become more compassionate and understanding of what patients experience and need to know. Sometimes they learn that procedures are done more for the staff's convenience than for the benefit of the patient. Illness alters a person's perspective, often making her more diplomatic, more empathetic. The situation is similar to that of tourists visiting a foreign country who meet people from their home state. They are able to achieve rapport quickly because of their perception that they have shared common experiences.

Being the recipient of care can inspire creative solutions to previously rigid systems. Consider the story of Dianne Martz, president and CEO of Hemophilia Health Service in Nashville, Tennessee (Snow, 1996). When her son was born with hemophilia, she was told that she could expect to make frequent trips to the hospital or to a federally funded treatment center for infusions of blood-clotting proteins. Wanting her son and others to have a healthy and normal life, she designed her company so that patients have supplies and medications delivered to their homes, where they can self-infuse the proteins. The company provides monitoring via telephone and home visits.

Whenever you or one of your staff members are patients at another practice or organization, evaluate the quality of service and follow-up attention you receive before, during, and after your visit. How soon do you receive test results, and how are they communicated? How is billing handled?

One of the advantages of being a patient or simulating the patient experience is that it reminds you to consider the patient's perspective in your organizational decisions. Then, before you purchase an automated patient registration system, for example, you will think about whether the new system will cost you an opportunity to establish rapport with patients.

Use Your Patients' Expertise

Do not overlook the expertise of patients. Bringing patients into the design process is a means of addressing patient expectations proactively. Whether you are evaluating brochures, voice mail scripts, or potential employees, patients can give you invaluable perspective that will almost always result in a better product or an improved service.

What do patients want that you can't give them? Keep a wish list, and monitor how other practices are responding to similar requests. What do patients need when the unexpected happens? Guests at resorts don't expect rain, so when it rains, world-class hotels have umbrellas on hand for guests' use. An obstetrical center that specialized in high-risk deliveries provided disposable cameras for patients who arrived unprepared. Armstrong Ambulance in Arlington, Massachusetts, always carries socks for patients whose families are too anxious to think of putting socks on a patient's feet before the ambulance arrives.

Listen carefully when patients speak about other organizations. A patient might mention how convenient it is to wait for a call from the children's pediatrician: "Robert's pediatrician now has call-in and call-back hours. You can call between 7:00 and 8:00 A.M. and speak to her within just a few minutes. And if you call later in the day, she will call you back between 4:00 and 5:00 P.M. It's a great time saver for me."

Encourage employees to capture and act on new ideas from patients. Some large companies keep notes on the comments customers make when they place orders, sharing those comments with all employees as a means of generating the greatest number of suggestions for improvement or new ideas. One staff member heard a patient say, "Well, the least Dr. Ohta could do is apologize, since she didn't show up for the appointment I was supposed to have last week." The staff member began clipping a note to charts of patients whose appointments were canceled when the obstetrician was called to a delivery. This simple and thoughtful act reminded the physician to apologize for inconveniencing the patient when they next spoke.

Successful companies always monitor the pulse of their communities. Considering that women are key decision makers regarding medical care, it makes sense to read the local women's press—especially those publications that focus on health care issues. You may discover that the community is learning to expect evening and weekend hours and that if an organization does not offer those hours, it is perceived as inflexible or outdated. What have the local media identified as the most significant health needs and barriers to care in your community? What can you do to change any negative situation for patients in your practice?

View Vendors as Consultants to Your Practice

Instead of viewing managed care and pharmaceutical representatives as time stealers, consider them industry experts who can share information about how changes in their businesses will affect your future. They can also provide you with competitive information about how other practices in their sales region are improving services for patients.

Anticipate Needs

Just before takeoff of a Florida-bound jet, the flight attendant, anticipating needs, walked down the aisle with a tray of tiny cups, asking, "Does anyone else need to take their pills?"

Recently, I took a 6:30 A.M. flight from Myrtle Beach, South Carolina, to Atlanta, Georgia. Because the duration of the flight was less than an hour, no food was served. As we exited the plane, the flight attendant handed each of the passengers a single breath mint and said, "Thanks for flying with us." The reaction of the passengers was, "Just what I needed!" Would something as simple as a mint help a patient waiting to see an ophthalmologist or ENT specialist?

Anticipating a patient's need and offering a solution even before he knows he has the need creates patient loyalty.

Make Every Trip a Field Trip

Every organization you visit or do business with has the potential to provide you with transferable ideas. Peter Drucker tells his clients that they must spend a few weeks every year outside their business if they want to grow their companies (Lenzner and Johnson, 1997).

Formal analysis of best practices would require you to find several companies that excel in a process you are interested in. To identify such companies, read business and trade publications faithfully. Companies that have won the Malcolm Baldrige Award agree to share their best practices with others. Leading companies such as FedEx, Ritz Carlton, Motorola, Saturn, and USAA have well-organized programs that are open to anyone to attend. At FedEx, participants visit the central Memphis hub at midnight to observe how packages are routed to their correct destinations. The following day includes a visit to the FedEx call center and meetings with managers about the company's guiding principles. A physician interested in best practices for tracking patient test results would benefit from seeing how FedEx tracks a million packages a day. Disney University hosts seminars on topics such as leadership, quality service, and people management. Motorola provides seminars on how it manages its Six Sigma quality culture and total customer satisfaction processes. In Spring Hill, Tennessee, visitors tour the Saturn plant and attend a workshop on high-performance productivity. At USAA in San Antonio, Texas, participants walk through the largest office building in the world and learn about the company's employee-friendly culture.

Do not limit your research to large companies. Mobil Oil, a company with 37,000 employees and revenues of more than $75 billion dollars in 1996, benchmarks with the West Concord, Massachusetts, 5 & 10, a store with fourteen employees and revenues of $1 million—to learn how to solve customer problems (Hofman, 1997).

The advantage of learning from businesses outside of health care is that you are obliged to be more creative in finding ways to incorporate their successes in your practice. You have to think differently. Consultants who specialize in organizational change like to say that if what you *think* remains the same, what you *do* will be difficult to change. Thinking creatively enables you to develop innovations that make your organization unique.

Some executives take every opportunity they can to ask people about their experiences in their industry. Sitting next to someone on a plane or meeting someone at a social function gives you an opportunity to hear the views of people who might be similar to your patients.

Consider an organization with which you enjoy doing business. What is it about the organization that makes you feel the way you do? Our customer experiences are often transferable to the practice. A staff member called a health club to ask about aerobics classes and said that she was self-conscious about her weight. "You won't be bringing in anything we haven't seen before," the receptionist reassured her. The practice team agreed that the same kind of reassurance would be helpful to patients who expressed reluctance about asking questions.

Successful companies concentrate on making everything easy for the customer. What makes it easier for patients to be patients? Where do patients get stuck in your system? Are there ways to expedite the registration process, perhaps with at-home preregistration? If you require patients to move from one area to another in an examining gown, could you instead provide a bathrobe to wear? One outpatient laboratory had no place except the floor for patients to place their handbags and coats while giving a urine specimen. An employee noted the design and manufacturer of shelving and coathooks while using the restroom at the airport.

Are there ways to make negative experiences more palatable? Some grocery stores offer free samples whenever long lines form at the cash registers. A pantyhose manufacturer, realizing that its customers hated buying and wearing pantyhose, added a motivational quotation to every package. In retail, one obstacle in ordering from catalogues is that returning merchandise is a nuisance. Omaha Steaks does not require customers who are dissatisfied with their steaks to return them in order to obtain a replacement or refund. The replacement or refund is given at the customer's request, no questions asked. Nordstrom gives customers a FedEx shipping label and a toll-free number to arrange for free pick-up of merchandise the customer wants to return. A restaurant that catered to business travelers noticed that solo diners often brought books to the dinner table but that the subdued lighting of the restaurant made reading difficult. They replaced the candles at some tables with small reading lamps. A medical practice that catered to businesswomen installed telephones in the reception area and examination rooms to enable patients to do two things at once.

There are endless opportunities to learn from other industries—both formally and informally. New York Hospital asked managers in the human resources, building services, food and nutrition, and admitting departments to meet with their counterparts at the Pierre Hotel. They came away with concrete strategies for improving service, such as keeping employee areas as clean as the rest of the hospital, developing mentoring programs to pair new employees with veterans, and improving their hiring practices (Montague, 1995b).

An organization that excels at helping its customers know what to expect is McDonald's. Even a person who has never eaten at a McDonald's can describe walking up to a counter, giving an order to a friendly face, receiving the meal on a tray, and taking it to a table. McDonald's uses advertising to teach people how their system works. Knowledge of what to expect is why visitors to Ellsworth, Maine, will go to McDonald's for a lobster roll instead of an attractive-looking restaurant that might turn out to be the best or the worst in the area.

When the *New York Times* asked, "Who is the best restaurateur in America?" (Drucker, 1996, p. 45) the answer was McDonald's, because "McDonald's has no bad tables, there's no tipping and the French fries are always a quarter-inch square. The customer wants no surprises and there aren't any, . . . the restaurant with none of the usual complications of a restaurant." McDonald's serves meat, potatoes, and beverages, items that are available almost everywhere. It's the packaging and the consistency of the experience that distinguishes McDonald's.

If you are part of a health care system and have successfully promoted it as an integrated delivery system, patients will expect that care received in one component of the network will be consistent with that received in other network facilities. Consistent service within the system is difficult to achieve, considering how hard it is to achieve even within any one practice. It is important that a system standardize policies and ensure that information is immediately available at all locations where patient care is provided. Many large systems are unaware of the patients they share, so a centralized database is essential. One-time registration and availability of registration and clinical information across the system are expected by today's pressured and confused patients. Consistency of service across various components of a health care system is very important in meeting expectations created by system advertising.

Consider Guarantees

"Guaranteed or your money back." Of course, you would never say such a thing to a patient. Or would you? Do you ever offer off-the-cuff guarantees, such as, "We'll take care of everything," or, "After the surgery, you'll be better than new"? Such statements can create expectations that might be impossible for you to meet.

Guarantee programs must be carefully crafted so as not to create unrealistic expectations for patients. Christopher Hart (1993), author of *Extraordinary Guarantees*, believes there are four components to an effective guarantee. Guarantees must be

1. Easy to understand
2. Easy to communicate

3. Meaningful and credible

4. Hassle free

In health care, there are two types of guarantee programs: medical and service. Organizations offering medical guarantee programs must be conscientious about informed consent. Medical guarantee programs are naturally more difficult to devise and thus are often loaded with fine-print exceptions. At a Minnesota fertility clinic (Gianelli, 1995), couples were promised, "Pregnancy or your money back." The program promised to refund all but $2,000 of prepaid fees if three attempts at in-vitro fertilization failed to achieve a viable pregnancy within eighteen months. Critics of the program pointed out that the warranty program was open only to couples in which the woman was thirty-five years old or younger and had normal uterine and ovarian functions, and the man had at least some sperm in his semen—the couples least likely to need the warranty.

Blue Cross and Blue Shield of Massachusetts took a different approach with a service guarantee instituted at their ten freestanding health centers. They developed a simple process by which patients could invoke the service guarantee when service did not meet their expectations. The information obtained by the health centers whenever the service guarantee was invoked provided workable advice. "It gives us information to know how to improve quickly," said Matt Kelliher, president of Status One Health Systems. "We see this as patients' prescription to us." Kelliher says that the program has increased patient loyalty and retention.

Indeed, the Blue Cross program is very specific about the commitment to patients: "We will see you when you feel you need to be seen, avoid inconvenient delays in serving you, treat you in a competent, compassionate and friendly way, listen to you and understand your needs, care for you as a person and as our patient and provide you with information to help you maintain or improve your health and lifestyle." The guarantee states: "If, as a patient in our health center, you are not completely satisfied that these services meet our commitment, please tell us immediately. We will strive to resolve the problem and promptly forward you your next month's health insurance payment. The amount we forward to you will be equal to the value or approximate value of the monthly individual employee contribution."

Internal resistance to the idea of guarantees is common. Physicians and staff fear that untrustworthy patients will abuse the system by filing false complaints. At Blue Cross, one physician angrily suggested that any patient who was not fully satisfied after three visits could receive a free sigmoidoscopy. Kelliher was careful to design the program so that Blue Cross guaranteed only what its representatives said it would do. If a patient claimed, "My doctor didn't order the CAT scan I needed," the company's response would be that the doctor never said he or she would order the scan. But if a patient invokes the service guarantee because he is unhappy with service, administrators do not take exception—they accept the patient's perspective. However, if a patient invokes the guarantee three months in a row, the issues he raises are reviewed. If it is felt that the patient is abusing the program, Kelliher contacts the patient and discusses whether the patient's expectations are unrealistic (Kelliher, 1997).

Most service guarantee programs look for quantifiable criteria against which to measure invoking the guarantee. Car dealers, for example, can measure whether appointments are available within one day, whether an order was written up within four minutes, whether the car was ready at the agreed-upon time, and whether a thorough explanation of the charges and specific work done was provided. After hiring mystery patients to seek care for headaches at their hospitals, Columbia HCA began offering guarantees that patients would be seen within thirty minutes or their care would be free. The small print was extensive: the clock didn't start ticking until the registration forms were filled out; the patient had to request a refund within two business days; and the guarantee applied only to the hospital and emergency physician's charges, not lab tests, X rays, or care by any specialists.

The benefits of guarantee programs include the following:

Guarantees convince some customers that the product or service is of high quality. Lisa Ford (1996) believes that guarantees have the greatest impact when (1) the price of service is high, (2) the industry has a bad image, or (3) customers are unfamiliar with the product or service.

Guarantees can result in increased revenues. At Marriott hotels, managers found that a frequent complaint was the amount of time it took for guests to receive their breakfast from room service. In 1985, the company instituted a program that guaranteed delivery of breakfast within five minutes of the time requested by the guest. Breakfast room service volume jumped by 25 percent (Bowles and Hammond, 1991, p. 70). At the Robert Wood Johnson Hospital in New Jersey, an emergency department service guarantee program promised that patients would be seen by a nurse within fifteen minutes and by a physician within thirty minutes. During the first five months of the program, sixteen thousand patients were seen and only one asked for money back. The emergency department has doubled in size ("Hospital Stands Behind Promise . . . ," 1995).

Guarantees can help retain customers. In 1991, Xerox analyzed 480,000 customers to determine how satisfied they were with the company's products and services. The company found that the "very satisfied" customers were six times more likely than the merely "satisfied" to buy more Xerox equipment. Xerox set out to increase the percentage of very satisfied customers by upgrading service levels and guaranteeing customer satisfaction (Heskett and others, 1994). Patient retention was a goal of the Blue Cross service guarantee program. Retention of those who invoked the service guarantee was an astounding 97 percent.

Guarantees create accountability. In praising the idea of medical guarantees, Stephen Cohen (1996, p. 12) has said, "The idea of accountability is attractive. And there are some things that the layman is qualified to judge—like compassion, kindness and dedication. Perhaps if doctors were financially accountable for their performance in these areas, there would be more empathetic doctors and more satisfied patients."

Guarantees can help build image. When FedEx makes good on a high-profile guarantee, it gives the company another chance to emphasize the benefit of its service. When actress Demi Moore was filming a movie and ordered some exercise equipment that arrived twelve hours late, FedEx canceled the $1,000 shipping fee. A spokeswoman for FedEx said, "Any customer can request a refund if a shipment is even one minute late" (Fink, 1996, p. 28). The benefit to existing and potential customers of FedEx was thus reinforced.

Study Exceptional Companies

Information is readily available about what exceptional companies have done to create and maintain success. Smith & Hawken, for instance, credits much of its success to simple service guidelines. In his book *Growing a Business*, Paul Hawken (1987) discusses the following employee guidelines in detail:

- Create legendary customer service.

- You are the customer—put yourself in the customer's position.

- You are the company. Employees don't need permission to be considerate.

- If it doesn't feel right, make it right.

- Do it yourself. Employees can take a customer service transaction from start to finish, making the employee's job more interesting.

- When in doubt, ask.

- A mistake is a chance to improve the company with better products, cost savings, new ideas, and better service.

Some best practices relate to simple consistency. Ritz Carlton has three steps of service (Barksy, 1995, p. 35):

1. A warm greeting in which the guest's name is used

2. Anticipation of and compliance with the guest's needs

3. A warm farewell, again using the guest's name if possible

The L. L. Bean customer satisfaction vision can give you a focus for discussion with your staff. "We understand our customers' needs. We meet those needs in a manner that distinguishes us from our competition and fosters a lifetime relationship with our company. We maintain a motivating, customer-focused environment that encourages individual commitment to continuous improvement and perpetuates a legendary reputation for customer satisfaction in which every employee feels personally vested." How do you foster a lifetime relationship with patients?

Rather than evaluating performance as a result of complaints or crises, successful teams make performance assessment part of their daily life. For years, sports teams have videotaped their games in order to critique them later. FedEx leadership meets every morning to review the prior day's performance. Everyone is expected to be there, on time, no excuses accepted. Lessons learned are exchanged with the expectation that people will put what they have learned into use to improve their operations (Ligos, 1997). Motorola has a half-hour meeting every day at 8:00 A.M. to communicate problems from the previous twenty-four hours that need to be addressed in the next twenty-four.

News coverage of successful companies can be used to guide staff discussions. The *Wall Street Journal* published a story about No Kidding, a Massachusetts toy store that has developed a very loyal clientele. The store creates loyalty by wrapping gifts at no charge; accepting returns without receipts; making donations to local schools; and extending discounts to teachers, grandparents, and contributors to public television (Pereira, 1996). Could some of these strategies be transferable to your practice?

Network

Belonging to professional groups is an opportunity to gain understanding of how other practices operate, become aware of others' best practices, and build a network of contacts. Before beginning a project, practice managers can solicit lessons learned from other practice managers to increase awareness of strategies that worked well and those that did not. Networking provides the benefits of smoother implementation, increased productivity, not having to reinvent the wheel, and elimination of errors and rework. Companies with multiple locations often have *twinning* programs, which take a staff member from one location and switch him with an employee in a similar position at another location. These kinds of strategies lead to the adoption of best practices and to enhanced service consistency.

◆ ◆ ◆ ◆ ◆ ◆

Encourage every staff member to participate in best practice initiatives. Do not let staff become discouraged if an idea isn't used or doesn't work out well. General Electric gives an award for the best *unused* employee suggestion. And be sure to celebrate the successes that improved quality or achieved patient or employee satisfaction.

Part IV

. . . .

Responding to Unmet Expectations

13

Complaints

Hot heads and cold hearts never solved anything.
                                        Billy Graham

Complaints. They will find you. It's inevitable that on occasion, schedules will go awry, patients will misinterpret efficiency for insensitivity, or patient expectations will not be met, and complaints will be the result. This chapter addresses obstacles to effective complaint handling, a ten-step process for handling complaints, and some strategies for dealing with patients' number-one complaint—waiting.

A complaint can be based on a failure to meet a patient's realistic or unrealistic expectations. When a patient complains, he is, at the outset, expressing a need for you to help him resolve a problem. He is saying, in effect, "Help. I want this relationship to continue, but I need you to help me." Patients who complain are actually more loyal than those who are dissatisfied but say nothing.

Americans as Healthcare Consumers: The Role of Quality Information, a national survey conducted by the Kaiser Family Foundation and Agency for Healthcare Policy and Research (1996) found that people are most interested in quality measures that emphasize patient experiences and satisfaction. Such items as how many complaints had been filed against physicians, the percentage of plan members who change plans because they are dissatisfied, and how patients rate their doctors were among the most important factors. Dealing with complaints at the earliest possible moment, often referred to as *service recovery*, is vital to achieving high ratings in health plan surveys. Willingness to resolve problems is a key driver of patient satisfaction that significantly affects a patient's desire to return and to refer other patients to you.

Ironic as it may sound, problems can create enduring relationships between people. Customer service experts believe that someone whose problem is resolved to his satisfaction is a more loyal customer than someone who has never had a problem at all.

Many Patients Would Rather Change Physicians Than Complain

A patient has been described as one who bears misery and pain without complaint. It is unfortunate that most patients don't complain when their expectations aren't met. Harvard Business School professor Theodore Levitt (1986) wrote in *The Marketing Imagination*, "One of the surest signs of a bad or declining relationship with a customer is an absence of complaints. Nobody is ever that satisfied, especially over an extended period of time. The customer is either not being candid or not being connected." Patients may not want to be perceived as "difficult" people. They may fear retaliation. They may not know to whom to complain. They may have complained in the past, without satisfaction. They may believe that complaining won't make a difference. Patients who say nothing to you will say plenty to others and may choose another physician. The writer Don Herold said, "Many doctors think that the patient has been cured, when he has merely quit in disgust." Preventing negative word of mouth requires listening for clues that patients are dissatisfied and then responding promptly to whatever their issues are.

Obstacles to Effective Complaint Handling

There are three common obstacles to effective complaint handling. The first is that physicians and staff do not know how to respond effectively to complaints. Although we know how we like to be treated when we have a complaint, few of us have had the opportunity to receive training in complaint handling. Is it any wonder that we often bumble through the complaint resolution process? We try to avoid "getting stuck with" complaints, preferring to dismiss them or trying to get rid of them as quickly as humanly possible—often passing the patient off to someone else. Organizations that excel in customer satisfaction provide companywide training so that whoever first learns of a complaint owns it until it is resolved—even if it's not her responsibility or involving her department. Training takes the focus of complaint handling away from defending the status quo or finding someone else to blame for the problem. In a patient-oriented practice, you won't find a staff member saying to a patient, "This is just my job. I'm doing what they told me to do. Talk to the doctor if you don't like it."

When an employee does not respond to a complaint in a professional manner, who does the patient get mad at? Certainly he gets mad at the employee but also at you and at the practice in general. Many companies measure the effectiveness of their complaint handling processes by measuring how many complaints are resolved during the initial contact or telephone call. If you want to achieve this kind of "once and done" approach in your practice, make it possible for everyone in the practice, not just front-line staff, to participate in training on complaint handling.

The second common obstacle to effective complaint handling is the tendency to delay responding in hope that the problem will resolve itself. The difficulty here is that even if the initial problem is fixed, you have caused a second problem by failing to get back to the patient. What is wrong may not be as important as what is done about it. A prompt response to a complaint is a key component of good service. Delay may cost you a patient. Research conducted by British Airways showed that 40 to 50 percent of customers who had complaints defected if it took longer than five days to respond (Weiser, 1995). As a result, the airline devotes resources to responding to complaining customers the same day. British Airways expects employees to respond *before* a customer writes a letter or makes a telephone call. William McDonough, senior vice president of J & H Marsh & McLennan, suggests that practices adopt a three-day turnaround time to resolve complaints (William McDonough, telephone interview with the author, 1997). Do not fall into the trap of establishing an elaborate system to resolve complaints. Writing a memo and waiting for a reply takes valuable time that can be better spent resolving the issue with the patient.

The third obstacle to effective complaint handling is a "mine is better" mentality. People have a very natural, ego-building desire to have the upper hand in situations. Children believe that their school is the best, their Dad's car is the best. Adults believe that their church is the best, that their political party is the best. You and your staff may believe that your way of doing things is the best. You want people to respect your knowledge, your authority, and your organization, and you may subconsciously view a complaint as a sign of disrespect. Although you want to be the best, be conscientious about not letting corporate culture get in the way of remembering what your mission is all about. If you do, you may not be open to ideas that can make your organization even better. One patient who spoke up about an issue of concern was dismissed with the following comment by the physician: "And where did you receive your medical degree?" If you view a complaint as an attack on your professionalism, your defensiveness will discourage complaints.

People are also defensive about complaints because so many complaints involve service rather than the product itself. According to Jon Anton (1996) of Purdue University, 68 percent of customers change products or suppliers because they had problems with customer service. Zagat, a company that surveys restaurants, found that over half of the complaints it receives about restaurants relate to service, whereas only 15 percent of complaints relate to food (Fabricant, 1996). Being prepared to respond to service complaints as competently as you do to physical complaints enables you to manage your relationships as effectively as you manage your patients' medical conditions.

How to Encourage Complaints

The best way to encourage complaints is to be approachable and genuinely receptive to them. It is important to identify small problems so that you can handle them while they are still small. Treating complaints as opportunities means that a patient's complaint is handled quickly. When you create a mind-set that complaints are something to be grateful for, you begin to see that they are actually unique opportunities to view service through your patients' eyes. Every dissatisfaction is an opportunity to differentiate yourself and your practice. Encourage staff members to think, "This is good. This is my chance to solve a problem and make someone's life better. This is my chance to make a difference, so I'm going to put myself in the patient's position while I listen to the complaint."

Staff members usually learn about problems before you do. Patients don't just pick up the telephone and call you with their evaluation of how an office visit went. They typically express their concerns to a staff member first, often before they leave the office. If you argue with staff members when they alert you to problems, you will discourage them from solving problems. Ten years later, staff members will encounter a problem and think, "Well, I did tell them about it, and they weren't concerned." All over America, employees are agreeing with customers who are dissatisfied with some aspect of the service they have received. "Yes, he's always late." Or worse, "Oh, you don't know the half of it." Has there been a hospital patient in the last decade who hasn't heard a staff member say, "Sorry, but we're short-staffed, you know."

Another way to encourage complaints is to make it easy for people to complain. One company, Intuit, gives some customers microcassette recorders, so that any time they get irritated they can simply press the record button and file their complaint (Lieber, 1997). In some hospitals, patients are given the name and telephone number of the CEO and the chief nursing officer upon admission. Many hospitals have installed hotlines that connect directly to the patient advocate or ombudsman.

Brook Run Family Physicians in Richmond, Virginia, prints the following information in the practice's brochure for patients: "When diagnosis and management are difficult, we will discuss the situation with you. We welcome the opportunity to include family members in the discussion. Some illnesses are difficult to evaluate and to treat. Frustrations and fears can be handled best if we discuss them frankly and work together toward your best possible health care."

You also encourage complaints when you let the patient know that you acted on his complaint or suggestion. This is a tremendous compliment to a patient.

Ten-Step Process for Responding to Complaints

The next section discusses in detail the ten steps to effective complaint handling. The list that follows summarizes these steps.

1. Watch for nonverbal clues of dissatisfaction.

2. Focus on the problem, not the patient's personality.

3. Recognize that the patient might be right.

4. Listen to the entire story, without interruption.

5. Demonstrate empathy.

6. Find some area of agreement.

7. Treat the patient as an individual.

8. Commit to take action.

9. Be clear about who will do what next.

10. Assure the patient of your desire for an ongoing relationship.

Step One: Watch for Nonverbal Clues of Dissatisfaction

Stay alert to signs that the patient or family is troubled. It takes only one incident of poor service to mar an otherwise exceptional relationship. Author Jim Rosenfield (1997) cites the "law of the 901st transaction." You can get it right 900 times, but if you make a mistake on the 901st, your future relationship still hinges on how you deal with the mistake. Be especially alert to the patient who responds to a question with a clipped "Fine." Be proactive about identifying problems. At California Pizza Kitchen restaurants, employees are taught clues to make sure that they spot unhappy customers as early as possible. Employees are advised that they should act immediately when they notice guests who are anxiously looking around, stacking their dishes, nervously tapping their silverware, negatively shaking their head, not eating their food, or asking for the check early (Thompson, 1997).

A patient who answers abruptly or whose tone of voice begins to rise or who crosses his arms while you are speaking may be providing clues that there is a concern that you need to address. Other clues include the patient's pausing or hesitating or stumbling over words.

Step Two: Focus on the Problem, Not the Patient's Personality

Avoid such thoughts as, "Oh, she is always cantankerous." Help staff give the patient the benefit of the doubt. Do they evaluate their own personalities in the same way? Many people are skilled at finding fault with others but can't see those same faults in themselves. For example, when the other person blows up, she's nasty; when we do it, it's righteous indignation. When he's set in his ways, he's obstinate; when we are, we're just being firm. When she sees flaws, she's picky; when we do, we possess excellent attention to detail.

Step Three: Recognize That the Patient Might Be Right

Approach the situation with the attitude that the patient could be right. It is easy to discount a patient's perspective, but sometimes the most unlikely things turn out to be true. At one hospital, a patient complained that bed bugs were biting her arms and legs. A physician dismissed her complaint, writing in the chart that the patient needed a psychiatric consult. While waiting for a physical therapy session, the patient looked at her chart and became angry when she saw the entry. As it turned out, the hospital was in fact experiencing a rash of bugs, and it ended up experiencing negative publicity too.

A patient complained to her physician that the phlebotomist was rough. The physician's initial inclination was to ignore the complaint. He decided, though, to ask the phlebotomist to draw blood from his arm and found that she was rough! He arranged for her to receive additional training, her technique improved, her patients were happier, and so was she.

Step Four: Listen to the Entire Story, Without Interruption

Lisa Ford (1996) says, "There is a difference between listening and waiting for your turn to speak." You cannot listen while you are talking. So do not interrupt, even if you can resolve the problem quickly. Listening gives you more information to work with when you do respond.

Step Five: Demonstrate Empathy

Take a moment to provide empathy before responding to the issue. As someone whose life's work is to devise solutions for problems, you may be naturally inclined to try to fix the problem quickly and be done with it. If problems are fixed by people with poor attitudes or without empathy, they may fix the problem but fail to fix the relationship. The patient may have received what he wanted, but without your empathy he may not feel that you cared. An indifferent attitude on the part of the listener often compounds a person's distress, so guard against insincere, programmed responses.

Reflective empathy is a connecting skill that helps you reduce repetitive statements by the patient, move toward a solution, and develop or maintain your relationship. Paraphrasing what the patient has said shows empathy and ensures that you understand what the person meant. Reflective empathy is the process of giving back understanding to the patient—whether or not you can give him what he actually wants. To reflect empathetically, begin by listening to the patient to determine the emotion that is driving the complaint. What is the problem costing the patient emotionally? Second, restate the meaning briefly, in an empathetic tone of voice. To start, try a phrase similar to these:

In other words, you're *afraid* that you won't be pain free after surgery.

You feel that it's *unfair* that insurance doesn't cover the total charge.

Your sense is that Dr. Taylor *promised* you the first appointment today.

It sounds as if you were *surprised* that the drug caused a headache.

When appropriate, you can validate your patient's feelings without agreeing, by saying something like, "If I experienced something like this, I'd be upset too." This kind of statement makes you an ally of the patient.

Third, when you have the patient's agreement that you understand the issue, proceed. Use a statement such as, "I can help you," to let the patient know you are on his side, but do not make promises you can't keep.

Step Six: Find Some Area of Agreement

If the patient thinks he has a problem, he has a problem. His perception is his reality. British Airways training focuses on helping staff members understand that if the company claims that events did not happen as the customer suggested, then the customer perceives that he is being called a liar. Resist the urge to disprove the patient's statement, even if you can. Find something that the person is right about. "You're right, Mr. Sullivan, things are not the same around here since Marie left. We miss her too." Fogging is a technique that you can use to find agreement in situations where the patient's remarks are exclusively critical. While the patient states his complaint, listen for any truth or logic in the situation. Point out the aspects of the complaint with which you do agree. For example, if a patient says, "You let the phone ring too long here," you might respond by saying, "You're right. The phone could be answered sooner." If the patient says, "You're too careless," you might respond, "You're probably right. I could be more careful." And, if the complaint is valid, apologize with sincerity. McDonough, of J & H Marsh & McLennan, says that apologizing for a problem is not an admission of liability, a concern many physicians struggle with when patients complain (William McDonough, telephone interview with the author, 1997).

Step Seven: Treat the Patient as an Individual

Some statements are verbal red flags to patients. Never say, "No one else has ever complained about this," or, "You're not our only patient, you know," or, "Everyone has to follow these rules."

When you put your patient on the defensive by using statements like these, he will be reluctant to approach you again. Or worse, the patient may consider your statements "fighting words" and retaliate by criticizing you to others, including the media.

On January 21, 1996, the front-page headline of the *Santa Fe New Mexican* read, "St. Vincent Form on Funeral Choices Angers Patient." What would make a patient so angry that the issue became headline news? The patient, who had been recently diagnosed with breast cancer, was upset to find forms in the hospital admission packet asking about her preferences for her funeral, obituary, and eulogy. The hospital's intent was to help patients make decisions ahead of time, in case they became too ill later on. The patient, whose daughter was a nurse at the hospital, went to administration to complain and was told that no other patients had complained about the forms. The hospital's response to the press, as reported in the headline story, was "Hospital says questions are standard, no other complaints registered" (p. 1).

In that same issue of the *Santa Fe New Mexican,* a lead story in the local section was titled "Competition Gets Clinic to Show Concern for Espanola." This story reported on a patient who went to the administrator of a kidney dialysis center in Santa Fe to request a satellite center for the patients living in the suburb of Espanola. The administrator dismissed the request, saying that all the other patients could drive to Santa Fe, so why couldn't that patient? The patient then approached a competitor and persuaded that organization to set up a satellite center. The first center then opened a clinic there as well.

One complaint may express the sentiments of other patients, so it's best to respond to each one in a serious and concerned manner. At Kent County Memorial Hospital in Warwick, Rhode Island, a patient complained about the hospital's tradition of playing Brahms's "Lullaby" each time a baby was delivered. The patient, who had suffered a miscarriage, heard the lullaby played over the intercom in her room and later felt that it was insensitive to patients in her situation. When she complained, the hospital spokeswoman gave this world-class response: "I am very distressed about Mrs. [patient's name]. I apologized to her and really felt awful. . . .

The hospital immediately decided to suspend it" ("Complaint Puts to Rest Maternity Room Lullaby," 1997, p. B11).

Step Eight: Make a Commitment to Take Action

Do not make assumptions about what your patients want. Ask, "What would make this right for you?" "What can we do to resolve this problem?" "What would satisfy you?" or, "What would you like me to do?" Then do something. If you can't give the patient exactly what he wants, give him *something*. Following through on a small promise is better than promising something you can't give and then failing to deliver. When a Delta Air Lines passenger wrote to the *New York Times* complaining about the way her baggage was inspected, a spokesperson for the airline responded as follows: "We apologize for any embarrassment [the customer] experienced. The safety and security of our customers, employees and facilities are a top priority. Yet Delta requires sensitivity and respect. We have contacted our security contractors and have identified how this situation might have been handled in a more considerate manner." Although they couldn't turn back time to reverse the embarrassment the customer felt, they validated her feelings and promised to do something to prevent the situation from happening again.

Step Nine: Be Clear About Who Will Do What Next

If you promise that you will take action, you must follow through or get back to the patient about the delay.

Step Ten: Assure the Patient of Your Desire for an Ongoing Relationship

This step is critically important if you want to preserve a relationship with your patient.

Occasionally, I arrive at a hotel to find that there is no record of my reservation. This causes me varying degrees of frustration, depending on the lateness of the hour and my own fatigue. One evening, everything was wrong. Despite my valid confirmation number, there was no record of my reservation, and all that was left was a smoking room. When I reacted in a less than charming manner, the clerk nodded in understanding (without agreeing, mind you) and said, "Mrs. Baker, I'm here until midnight. If there are problems I can work on, please call me and I'll try my best to resolve them." Her sincere offer to be of future assistance made me feel like a valued customer again.

Assuring a patient that you want the relationship to continue despite a problem lets the patient know that he can be himself. Saying something like, "Thank you for taking the time to tell me about your problem. I'm glad that we had this chance to talk, and I hope that if this ever occurs again, you'll let me know right away." The patient feels reassured that you want to continue the relationship and that he or she is still important to you. Unconditional acceptance is very memorable.

When you next handle a complaint, use the following checklist to assess how well you used the skills covered in this chapter.

- Did you speak in a calm tone of voice?

- Did you listen without interrupting?

- Did you indicate that you wanted to help?

- Did you promise only what you could deliver?

- Were you clear about who was going to do what next?

- Did you do what you said you would do?

- Did you check to see if the patient was satisfied?

Angry Patients

As a rule, patients are anxious. How does anxiety turn into anger? In his book *The Meaning of Anxiety*, Rollo May (1977, p. 230) wrote, "Anxiety and hostility are interrelated; one usually generates the other. First, anxiety gives rise to hostility. This can be under-stood in its simplest form in the fact that anxiety, with its con-comitant feelings of helplessness, isolation and conflict, is an exceedingly painful experience. One tends to be angry and resent-ful toward those responsible for placing him in a situation of pain." Anger can also be the result of stress caused by powerlessness or un-predictability. A person may believe that the release of tension through an angry outburst will help him regain control. Instead, it often backfires, as the recipient of the outburst becomes defensive or mirrors the angry patient's attitude.

A patient may also get angry when he feels he can't predict what is going to happen to him. You may not know the cause of his symp-toms. You may not know what his eventual course of treatment will be. Don't let that stop you from sharing what you do know. Simply knowing what will happen next can reduce patient anxiety.

Unmet expectations often lead to frustration, which increases anxiety and creates anger. Understanding the reason behind some-one's anger helps you deal with it more easily. A receptionist once told me about handing a registration form to a patient to complete and having the patient hand it back to her, saying, "I'd like you to fill it out." "Patients have to complete the form," she replied. The question of who would fill out the form was argued for another few moments, until the patient said, in a trembling voice, "Ma'am, I don't know how to read."

It is tempting to mirror the angry patient or to vent your own frustrations. At L. L. Bean, employees are taught that no one ever wins an argument with a customer. If you are prone to argue, remind yourself that you don't want to say anything that you will regret later. Consider how effective getting angry has been for you in the past. Whenever possible, delay any emotional response to the angry patient for a few moments or as long as it takes you to be calm. When someone is angry and says something outlandish, try letting the person's words echo back to him by saying nothing at all for a moment. If the patient doesn't modify his behavior, try asking in a low, calm tone of voice, "Excuse me, but I'd like to help. Would you mind telling me what you are getting out of treating me this way?"

When a patient isn't particularly pleasant or friendly, it is tempting to forget about building rapport with him and instead concentrate on completing the visit. Although you can't control a patient's behavior, you can control your response to that behavior. Your attitude determines how much stress you experience. It may help to keep in mind that this patient needs your kindness, perhaps even more than other patients do.

Angry patients may project their frustration onto the practice and that can be a good thing. The patient's reaching a point where he cannot bear his illness any longer and loses control can be an aid to his relinquishing unrealistic expectations, according to an Australian nursing study (Dewar and Morse, 1995).

The following are some tips for dealing with an angry person:

- Listen to the whole story without becoming defensive.

- Don't agree or disagree before you understand what the person means.

- If the patient is standing, invite him to sit down. Offer him something to drink. Make some change in physical setting.

- Touching an angry person may be perceived as an attack.

- Use the patient's name, in a calm tone of voice.

- If you know your patient well, use humor as appropriate, but don't ridicule.

- Don't gang up on the angry person. Don't involve someone else simply to support your position.

- Don't pass the person off to someone else.

- Don't mirror the patient's angry emotions. Do mirror

some of the patient's words to demonstrate empathy and understanding. If you slip into anger yourself, try saying this: "It wasn't my intention, but I have been arguing with you instead of listening to you. Would you please start again for me?"

- Try to find something the person is right about.

- Reverse roles: "If you were me, how would you handle this situation?"

Some angry people simply need to understand what's happening to them and have their frustration acknowledged. Before choosing to enter into an argument with an angry person, remember the old saying: "It's never good for a wise man to argue with a fool. Bystanders can't always tell the difference."

Difficult Patients or Patients with Difficulties?

Patients who are frequently anxious or who do not know what to expect may be uncooperative as a result. One study (Hall, Roter, Milburn, and Daltroy, 1996) found that physicians often engaged in less social conversation and agreed less with patients who were sicker than others and were frequently anxious. In turn, the sicker patients became even more distressed and angry. Thus the anxiety that patients feel can result in behaviors that you and your staff consider difficult. A British study (Sharpe and others, 1994) looked at why doctors found some patients "difficult to help." Difficult patients often had medically unexplained symptoms, coexisting social problems, and severe untreatable illnesses. The authors suggested that aligning the doctor's and patient's aims for care and improving the access to psychosocial care could improve the quality and cost-effectiveness of outpatient services.

Jeffrey Jackson of the Uniformed Services University of Health Sciences in Bethesda, Maryland, speaking at the 1997 annual meeting of the Society of General Internal Medicine, reported that patients with mood or anxiety disorders were twice as likely to be rated "difficult" by the physicians and were more likely to report unmet expectations with their office visits and to be dissatisfied with the care they received (Nidecker, 1997).

The Connecticut Medical Insurance Company advises its insureds that difficult patients will often respond to a combination of these eight techniques:

1. Pay attention to what the patient says. Difficult patients need to be taken seriously in order to be helped. Don't dispute the reality of their complaints. For these patients, their problems are serious and real.

   If you experience a negative emotional reaction to a difficult patient's responses or to their perception of illness—remember these patients are reacting in the best way available to them. Try to consider each difficult patient as a challenge to your diagnostic and therapeutic skills. Teach them other, more appropriate ways of reacting and responding to their problems.

2. Evaluate each new symptom before attempting to attribute the problem to a psychophysiologic reaction. Moving too quickly from the physical complaint to an emotional basis is usually met with resistance and hostility. Slowly elicit the psychological issues, and the patient will better understand their influence on the illness and be able to deal with them more appropriately.

3. Establish realistic, therapeutic goals, since a cure is usually an impossible end point. The goal may be to decrease the number of urgent telephone calls and unscheduled or emergency visits or to avoid

unnecessary hospitalizations or procedures. Help patients to increase their own sense of control over their symptoms.

4. Schedule appointments at regular intervals to avoid unscheduled visits contingent upon new or increased symptoms.

5. Avoid use of medications to treat minor depression, insomnia, anxiety and other minor associated somatic complaints. Treatment of these symptoms with medication rarely succeeds. Medications may increase and reinforce these patients' helplessness and lack of understanding of their symptoms.

6. Refer only if appropriate and then emphasize that this referral is not a dismissal. Follow-up with patients and continue to provide support after the referral.

7. Provide patients with a respectable "term" for their illness—a term to describe that illness to their family and friends. For example: abnormal peristaltic movements, increased muscular tension or anterior chest wall dysesthesia.

8. Control the agenda. Set the rules early in the therapeutic regimen. Reserve all but emergency complaints for the routine scheduled visits.

Accepting your inability to always totally cure a patient with somatic illness will help you avoid frustration and unachievable goals.

Difficult patients often have an intense desire to be part of a group. They are people whose own family members don't return their telephone calls. Help your patient feel part of your organization by letting him in on changes that will be taking place in the practice, especially any that are the result of concerns he brought to your attention. If encouraging him to belong doesn't work, remember that at least you don't have to take him home with you.

Another technique that has worked more than once is to let the difficult patient overhear you saying something nice about him. Or if this fails, let him hear you saying something especially nice about some other physician.

A wonderful example of dealing with a difficult person was submitted to *Medical Economics* by José L. Llinas of Florida, who told the story of a surgical instructor who was impossible to please. The instructor told one of his students to cut some sutures. Knowing that whatever he did would be wrong, the student said, "Yes sir, and shall I cut them too long or too short?" (Llinas, 1991, p. 135). Needless to say, this clever response is not appropriate for your demanding patient.

Difficult patients can be viewed as opportunities, because there is no competition for them. The difficult patient can help you improve your skills with other patients and may force you to make improvements in your style or practice that you might otherwise not recognize the need for.

> **Difficult patients can be viewed as opportunities, because there is no competition for them.**

Complaints About Waiting

"The patient waiting for you is counting your faults" is an old saying, and it tells us that people have never liked waiting. Women see doctors more often and are more likely to accompany others to medical visits. In the past, when fewer women worked outside the home, they expected to wait and, for the most part, accepted waiting as a normal part of a medical visit. Today, for many people in stressful jobs, time is more valuable than money because although anyone can get more money, no one gets more time. *The Rotarian* (August, 1996, p. 56), a publication of Rotary International, said it well: "Everyone's in such a hurry these days. In the era of the stagecoach, if you missed a coach you were content to wait for the next one to come in a day or two. Now, some people blow their tops if they miss one section of a revolving door." People want what they want when they want it. The World Wide Web has been called the World Wide Wait by consumers who can't tolerate a sixty-second wait for information.

An American Hospital Association and Picker Institute survey of 37,100 people found that 30 percent of respondents reported a problem with having to wait in doctors' offices or clinics; this was the most frequently mentioned problem associated with the outpatient setting (*Eye on Patients*, 1996).

The *Farmers' Almanac* has given a name to chronic tardiness in health care: CLS or Continual Late Syndrome (Appleby, 1996a). Its "Patients' Bill of Rights" recommends a discount or free consultation from any doctor who makes the same patient wait for three scheduled appointments.

Patients expect much more from office staff in terms of time and courtesy than they do from clinicians. However, as the length of time of waiting increases, patients expect far more from their physicians.

It may be that we hear more about patient dissatisfaction with waiting because patients are more willing to complain to someone indirectly. Is there a practice manager anywhere who hasn't listened to the complaint of a waiting patient who, moments later, was all smiles when he met with his physician? Even patients who do not express their dissatisfaction about waiting may be reluctant to refer friends and associates to you.

Many studies have shown a link between patient satisfaction and expectations and perceptions of waiting time. Typically, researchers find that patients are least satisfied when waiting times are longer than expected, are relatively satisfied when waiting times match expectations, and are most satisfied when waiting times are shorter than expected. Keeping patients informed about how long to expect to wait can be helpful. Other factors that influence patients' expectations regarding waiting time include age, employment status, prior experience, means of transportation, acuity of illness, duration of illness, insurance status, time of day, and whether the patient is accompanied by someone else. The Irish have a saying, "Two shorten the road"—a companion can make waiting more pleasant for a patient, unless that companion is short tempered about waiting and thus increases anxiety in the patient. The courteousness of staff members in providing an apology and explanation is very helpful in reducing the anxiety of those waiting.

At Harris Methodist Fort Worth Hospital, efforts were made to be more sensitive to patients, but satisfaction survey scores weren't rising accordingly (Appleby, 1996b). A team looked at the experience from the patient's perspective and instituted a new registration system to take patients directly to exam rooms and have encounter staff go to the patient. Waiting times have dropped from thirty-one minutes to four minutes, although the staff have to fill out information manually and then input data into the computer when they return to their desks. "I'm not going to run this ED based on the convenience of the staff," said the hospital's medical director of the emergency department. At-home preregistration of patients can save patients' time in the office. Newton-Wellesley Hospital in Newton, Massachusetts, offers patients Registration Express! service. Patients are given a brochure containing a perforated wallet card or Rolodex card. The card tells the patient what information will be needed when he calls to register and the times and the telephone number for the service.

Managing Expectations About Waiting

Mr. Visseray loves to visit his physician. It's really the highlight of his week, a social event because it's usually the only day that he leaves his home. He puts on his best suit and makes arrangements to arrive about an hour early. He waits and waits, and as he watches later arrivals being taken before him, he begins to get a bit agitated. What happened to first come, first served? Are those patients getting in quicker because the doctor or staff like them better? If he gets out of his chair to use the lavatory, will he miss his turn? He's reluctant to complain, but his perception is that he is being treated unfairly. For patients, unfair waiting seems longer. If this scenario is familiar to you, consider posting a sign that reads, "Patients are seen in order of appointment, not arrival." If your practice is organized so that patients are seen in order of check-in, you need to be conscientious about ensuring that the first come, first served policy is followed for all but the most unusual circumstances.

During an initial visit, take a moment to explain that there will be times when a patient has special needs that require more of the clinician's time, throwing the schedule off as a result. Very ill patients will sometimes take priority over patients waiting for routine care. If a practice offers obstetrics, there will be times when appointments will be delayed because a patient is in labor. You would think that patients would realize this on their own, but, as the old joke goes, if people were logical, men would ride sidesaddle.

Ruby Tuesday's restaurant in Greenville, South Carolina, kept two waiting lists for tables (Fromm and Schlesinger, 1993). One list was noticeably longer because patrons wanted to be waited on by a certain waitress. They didn't mind waiting longer for one of her tables because of the experience she created for them while they were there. You may have a similar situation if one of your physicians likes to take a lot of time with patients, resulting in a schedule that runs behind.

Most practices have physicians with different styles. Some physicians have schedules that patients can set their watches by. Other physicians never adhere to a schedule, choosing to be guided by an individual patient's physical and emotional needs. Letting patients know about the unique style of each physician can help the patient make a wiser choice that will match his own preferences. After all, the wait isn't as bad if you are choosing to wait.

Dansky and Miles (1997) found that informing patients about how long their wait would be and patients' having something to do during the wait were significant predictors of patient satisfaction.

Predictions offered about waiting time must be accurate and updated as promised. When a pilot tells passengers, "We will be circling the airport for twenty-five minutes," the plane must begin to land before that time, or the pilot must make another announcement before the twenty-five minutes have elapsed. At Disney theme parks, posted waits for admission to attractions are overestimated by a few minutes as a safety net against frustration.

A young mother was accompanying an older woman to a nine o'clock ophthalmology appointment. They had requested the first appointment of the day, because the younger woman had to meet her kindergartner's school bus at noon. At half past nine, more patients arrived, followed by another wave of patients at ten. The office staff person was shielded from those waiting by a wall and a door, and no one criticized her for this. At ten, the young mother went to see the receptionist to inquire about the delay. The receptionist responded that the doctor had not yet arrived. Returning to the waiting area, the other waiting patients began to discuss the fact that the doctor was always late for his appointments and that finding a waiting area full of patients was not unusual. At eleven, the patient was shown to an examination room. At eleven-thirty, the young mother left to meet the school bus, returning at twelve-thirty to collect the patient. The patient had spent three and a half hours in the office for a thirty-minute appointment. The young mother vowed to tell everyone she knew, including her primary care physicians, never to use that ophthalmologist.

Some practices will telephone patients when a physician or other clinician is running late in order to give the patient the option of coming later or rescheduling. Others welcome calls from patients to see if their physician is running on schedule. Both strategies are effective in managing waiting times.

Is it better to ask patients to wait in the reception area or in an exam room? Many adult patients tend to prefer the privacy of the exam room, if there are magazines there to review while they are waiting. Pediatric patients who are visiting for routine checkups prefer the activity and amusements of the reception area. Dansky and Miles (1997) recommend that patients not be moved quickly out of the reception area into an examination room only to experience a long wait, because the initial move can create expectations that care will be provided quickly. "A lengthy wait in the treatment room would then disconfirm those expectations, resulting in feelings of dissatisfaction, and, perhaps, anger and resentment" (p. 174).

Responding to complaints about waiting should begin with acknowledgment of the inconvenience. Let the patient know that it is acceptable to complain. If you are at fault, apologize. Do not mirror the patient's frustration with your own litany of pressures.

Four Strategies to Remove Dissatisfaction Caused by Waiting

There are several ways that you and your staff can prevent long waits or make unavoidable waits more tolerable.

Improve Scheduling

There are many scheduling systems and theories available to improve scheduling and minimize waits. Poor scheduling leads to crowded reception areas where some patients can infect others with dissatisfaction, not to mention illness. Poor scheduling can result in insufficient time for an adequate physical examination. One idea is to measure how long clinicians take with certain patients and under certain conditions. If you tell your receptionist to book thirty minutes for a physical exam but your physicals routinely take an hour, you are setting up your subsequent patients to be disappointed.

Give Patients an Opportunity to Do Two Things at Once

There are people who are happiest when they can do two things at once. In Lake Oswego, Oregon, a Chevron station offered mammograms while work was being done on patients' cars ("Gas Station Offers Mammograms," 1996). Some Nordstrom department stores offer walk-in mammography screening. SmartCare Medical Centers of South Bend, Indiana, established clinics in supermarkets, citing the convenient parking, easy access (no stairs), adjacent pharmacies, and motorized shopping carts. An endodontist has a manicurist on staff on Thursdays for complimentary manicures. A Washington, D.C., dry cleaner has photographs of single customers on his walls for matchmaking purposes ("Outliers," 1996).

Consider installing a telephone line for local telephone calls in your reception area. Business newspapers, journals, books, pens, paper, portable telephones, and a fax machine are amenities that you can offer to suit the preferences of your Type A patients.

The hotel industry is a rich source of knowledge about managing customers' experiences. For example, the hotel industry knows that its guests hate to wait for elevators. Research revealed that customers didn't mind waiting as much if they had a mirror to look into while they waited. That's why, at many major hotel chains, you'll see a mirror opposite the elevators and sometimes inside the elevator cab as well.

I told this story at a medical staff meeting in my area. Sometime later, I went to visit my gynecologist, who had moved to a new office building. The reception area had a lovely mirror. The floor-to-ceiling mirror in the lavatory was also lovely. In the examination room, there was a mirror behind the curtain. When my physician arrived, I said, "Doctor Browne, the mirrors are very nice, but do you think you're overdoing it just a little?"

With a twinkle in his eye, he replied, "The wait is the same, but the complaints have dropped so dramatically that the next time you come, there'll be a mirror on the ceiling."

Of course, attention to detail is important. Be sure, for example, the mirrors don't have messages on them saying, "Objects in mirror are larger than they appear."

Make Waiting More Comfortable

Comfort features such as soft music, relaxing chairs, tea, and aromatherapy can create a respite for waiting patients. If a relaxing atmosphere is what you would like to have for your patients, provide books for children rather than toys. A fish tank can be relaxing for adults and provide entertainment for children, especially those who aren't reading yet. At one practice, patients request appointments for tank cleaning afternoons, when the serviceman gives talks about the fish while doing his work.

Make Waiting Interesting and Fun

Some practices decorate for the holidays. One practice sets out a produce basket during the summer months so that patients with too much produce can share their surplus. Provide health information, such as injury prevention do's and don'ts, nutritional assessment questionnaires, reading recommendations, upcoming support group meeting dates and locations, and telephone numbers for hotlines on health issues. Crossword puzzle pads can be an interesting distraction for waiting patients and their companions.

Although people often do not like change, it is important that your office appear fresh and up-to-date. If you have taped music, change it regularly. Display fresh flowers, or live plants if you can keep them alive. Decorate the walls with exhibits of local artists and photographers; paint the crown moldings; change the lighting. Waiting is an unmined opportunity for many health care organizations. It's the one part of the visit that can be fun. Are your patients having more fun than they used to?

Nine Ways to Win the Waiting Game

1. Make a good first impression. This is the moment for smiles to be their brightest and warm personalities to be most evident. A welcoming receptionist can be the most pleasant part of a medical visit. Hire the smile and teach the skills.

2. Keep your reception area spotless and comfortable. Check the area several times a day to organize magazines and wipe up spills. Use single-seat chairs. Rocking chairs are nice, especially in obstetric or pediatric settings. Replace shabby or worn furniture as soon as possible.

3. Provide appropriate reading material. Subscribe to a variety of magazines written for a range of audiences. Avoid magazine collections that reflect a lavish lifestyle or only the physician's interests. A daily newspaper is also a good idea. One physician subscribes to *Hello*, the British version of *People*. His patients enjoy it because they don't read it anywhere else. Consider using a sign reading, "Please feel free to take home any magazine that is more than four months old." Another practice has a nice collection of cookbooks and provides cards for copying recipes. Humor books can be very entertaining, especially for patients who are anxious.

4. Establish a budget for flowers, individually wrapped mints, and other amenities. Some practices set up a coffee pot or a water cooler. Consider providing small bottles of water to drink while patients wait. Patients will tell others about your healthful generosity.

5. Provide relaxing distractions. Consider providing stationery, pens, and stamps for writing letters. An Etch-a-Sketch is a quiet, easy-to-clean toy for all ages. Music can be used to mask undesirable sounds, but audience analysis is critical when choosing a radio station. Avoid rock stations. Classical music is usually a good choice.

6. Accentuate the positive. Instead of *waiting room*, use the term *reception area*, to show that it's not just a holding area but a place designed for your visitor's comfort.

7. Borrow the patient's perspective. Walk in your own front door before office hours and sit quietly in the reception area for twenty minutes. What do you see, feel, hear, and smell? Is the chair comfortable for a twenty-minute wait? Is the wallpaper peeling? Do you feel any drafts, or is the sun beating in too strongly? Does the room smell fresh? Are the plants healthy? Can you overhear office staff conversations, perhaps even

conversations a patient shouldn't hear? You may be surprised at what you notice.

8. Keep patients informed. Explain all delays. Offer to reschedule if the wait will be long. Offer use of the telephone for waiting patients.

9. Apologize for delays. Let patients know how important their time is. Some practices offer discounted bills, restaurant coupons, or gift certificates to patients subjected to excessive waits.

Whoever Said the Customer Is Always Right Didn't Work in Health Care

I live in Connecticut near the Stew Leonard's grocery store. As you enter the store, you see, "Rule #1: The Customer Is Always Right," etched in a huge boulder. Next to that boulder is another, which reads, "Rule #2: If the customer is ever wrong, reread Rule #1."

Those rules work well at grocery stores. The folks at Stew Leonard's can make things right with a customer by replacing a pork roast or offering a gift certificate. But in medicine, it's very different. Your patient may want a medication that's contraindicated for him. He may want surgery because his brother had it or his insurance will cover it. He may arrive on the wrong day for his appointment and demand to be seen immediately.

When you can't give a patient what he wants, find out why he wants it. His explanation will provide valuable information to use in managing his expectations.

What does the patient really need? What is the best solution you can provide? For example, a patient who becomes angry with you because you won't perform the surgery that worked so well for his brother needs information. The patient who wants a prescription for Prozac because all his coworkers are feeling happy may need counseling, a stress reduction program, or an employee assistance program.

When the patient is wrong but you are going to take care of the problem anyway, you might as well be nice about it. Let's go back to the classic example of the patient who arrives a day early for his appointment. He says the appointment was scheduled for Tuesday; you say Wednesday, but you'll fit him in. Members of the team think that they are doing him a favor by reminding the patient that they are accommodating him, but all he's thinking is, "They made the mistake, and now they're trying to make me feel guilty."

If conflict exists because both you and your patient believe "I'm right—the other person is wrong" and you feel that you have reached an impasse in trying to resolve the situation, consider trying this: say to the patient, "I'd like to see if I understand your point of view. I'd like to repeat back what you've told me so that you can correct me if I've misunderstood something. Then I'd like you to tell me what you think I'm saying."

What should you do when your patient is wrong? Borrow a strategy from the Disney Corporation ("The Disney Approach to Quality Service," 1996). Disney says that it hopes its guests will always be right, but in the event that a guest is wrong, a cast member should let the guest be wrong with dignity. Speaking to the patient in a calm and understanding tone of voice, not proving the patient wrong in front of others, and not ridiculing the patient are a few ways to do this.

Tying Complaints to Future Improvements

Unpleasant though it may be, keep a record of complaints. FedEx has catalogued customer complaints since the early 1980s. The company refers to the process as the "hierarchy of horrors" and uses it to gain insight into customer expectations and disappointments. FedEx learned that different problems had varying impact on customers. For example, a damaged package was of greater concern than a late package. Using complaint data, FedEx was able to define twelve indicators and develop a measurement system to monitor prevention of those problems (*Blueprints for Service Quality*, 1994).

Establish a complaint log so that solutions receive ongoing attention. What are the key problems or complaints? Which problems do the most damage? Are there any trends? Analyze why the problem occurs and then identify improvements to eliminate the problem or to reduce its size or impact. For example, if parking will be a problem or if the reception area is being renovated, let patients know when they are making an appointment. Outside the South Station Tunnel in Boston, construction managers posted a sign for detoured commuters that read, "Rome wasn't built in a day. If it were, we'd have hired their contractor."

Do not set up elaborate resolution channels that take time away from responding to patients. Simply keep a list of problems that patients present to you and your staff. You may not be able to do anything with the seemingly unresolvable problems, but keep them on the list anyway. When a patient says, "I wish I didn't have to go over to the bad section of town for that test," that's a problem that could be an opportunity down the road. Denis Waitley (1995, p. 26) writes, "Before Fred Smith visualized Federal Express, people didn't consider the lack of an overnight express service a national problem. They simply thought, 'I'm in trouble. This package is supposed to be on Smither's desk in Denver tomorrow. I sure wish there was some way of getting it there by then.'"

· · · · · · · ·

Success is linked to the ability to solve problems and handle complaints. Tom Peters (1994) tells companies that the glowing letters are for the problem solvers—the people who can cope with the unexpected, who can see two sides of an issue, and who focus on answering the needs of the customer.

Answering the needs of patients who are angry or upset isn't always easy. Remember the old adage: "Try to do to others as you would have them do to you, and do not be discouraged if they fail sometimes. It is much better that they should fail than you should."

Although complaint handling requires skill and patience, it can also be among the most rewarding of your patient interactions. Patients who are well treated after having a complaint feel that you were there when they needed you.

14

Patient Follow-Through

Some men have thousands of reasons why they can-
not do what they want to do, when all they need is
one reason why they can.

Willis A. Whitney

One of the great frustrations of medicine is that a patient's outcome often depends on his ability or willingness to follow
through with the agreed-upon treatment plan. This chapter addresses some of the reasons why patients don't follow through and
identifies strategies for encouraging them to do so.

In his autobiography, *Only When I Laugh*, Robert Clifford (1982,
p. 79) facetiously expressed his frustration this way: "If anyone won-
ders what has soured the milk of doctors' kindness . . . wonder no
more. This is it: Patients of old were respectful of their doctor's feelings. They were careful not to behave in any manner that might put
her off her feed, such as questioning her judgement or failing to respond to her treatments. . . . In the interaction between the doctor
and the patient, it was the patient's job to get better and it was doctor's job to get the credit." Those days, if they ever existed, are gone
forever, along with the days of keeping the patient in the hospital
until every test has been tried or completed. Considering the
nonexistent hospital stays and many cost containment measures

instituted by managed care, patients have much greater responsibility for their actions. For patients to be successful, you have to give them information and motivation along with the freedom and responsibility to manage their care.

Patients want to know what to expect. They ask such questions as, "What is going to happen to me in the future?" or, "Do you think I'll get cancer?" When a patient wants you to predict the future, you have an excellent opportunity to explain how his own initiative can influence his future health status.

Why Patients Don't Follow Through

Some patients fail to follow through with their treatment plan because they do not want to get well. They want attention or have a desire to feel nurtured. They may be seeking relief from responsibility or trying to punish someone. Patients with chronic illnesses may not be perceiving adequate benefit from follow-through. Depression also may affect compliance (Katon and others, 1997).

For many patients, the more costly or complex the regimen and the longer it must be followed, the less likely they will be to follow through. Patients are also less likely to follow through when they believe that doing so will negatively affect their appearance—for example, some people take less insulin than prescribed in order to prevent weight gain.

Encouraging Patient Follow-Through

When developing and discussing a treatment plan with your patient, consider the following strategies to encourage compliance.

Explain Your Rationale

It's not enough to tell some patients what to do; you also have to tell them why they should do it. Explaining why something is important gives meaning to the change you expect of your patient.

The patient who understands the consequences of not following your advice is more likely to follow through.

In 1989, I needed back surgery. I had tremendous trust and confidence in my neurosurgeon. On the day of my discharge from the hospital, he sat on my bed and said, "Susan, I'll see you in a week to take out your stitches. Until then, don't vacuum, don't lift anything heavier than a piece of paper, and don't drive a car." My response was "OK, OK, OK." Six days later, someone called from his office and asked if I wanted to come that day for removal of the stitches. Would I? I hopped right into the car and drove ten miles to his office.

At the time, the neurosurgeon shared reception space with an ophthalmology practice. Standing at the reception desk was an older man waiting for his appointment with the ophthalmologist. He was telling the receptionist that he had had great trouble finding a cab to bring him to the office. I recognized the man as a former hospital patient and knew that he lived directly across the street from the hospital. I introduced myself to him and offered to drive him home if he wished.

My physician removed the stitches and ended the visit by saying, "Susan, you're doing great. I'll see you in three weeks, but until then, don't drive a car." I said "OK," walked out to the reception area, and asked the older gentleman if he was ready to leave.

We got into my car, in a very crowded parking lot, and I began to back the car out of its space. The car began traveling in reverse at a very high speed, and the harder I tried to step on what I *thought* was the brake, the faster it went. Mercifully, the car came to a stop without injuring anyone or anything. I looked at my passenger. "I'm not sure what to do now," I said in a trembling voice. "Well, I think I'll get out of the car," was his reply.

I learned from that experience that even patients who trust their physicians may think they know better if they are simply given instructions without a rationale. Had I known the implications of driving so soon after surgery, I would not have been behind the wheel

of my car that day. "Because I said so" is not a message that works
with patients who think it is perfectly rational to ignore a physician's advice.

Encourage Questions

No matter what you say or how you say it, your patient may not be
listening or understanding what you mean. Therefore, it is important that you create an atmosphere in which patients feel comfortable asking questions. You can create such an atmosphere by being
on the same physical level with the patient, making significant eye
contact, and asking, "What questions do you have?" or, "What concerns do you have?" Encouraging your patient to repeat or paraphrase what you say is also important.

Researchers at the University of Kansas School of Medicine
found that hospital patients had far less understanding than physicians thought they did. Physicians believed that 95 percent of their
patients knew when to resume normal activities, but only 58 percent of the surveyed patients agreed. The researchers recommended
targeted discussions, telephone follow-ups, and written reminders
as strategies to improve communication (Calkins and others,
1997).

Think about how you communicate. A study of older patients'
satisfaction with ambulatory care and compliance (Linn, Linn, and
Stein, 1982) found that satisfaction with care was correlated significantly with compliance and that satisfaction was associated with
the physician's expectations for improvement. Will your patient respond better if you explain that a medication works for 80 percent
of patients than if you say it doesn't work for 20 percent of patients?

Provide Written Information

Patient instruction sheets are often available from your professional
society or are fairly easy to prepare. They improve patient follow-
through, as patients often are thinking about the last instruction
you gave them or whether they can get to the pharmacy on time,

and may not remember your instructions. Even when they try to listen, anxiety can prevent them from recalling your advice later. With written information, patients can review your instructions at their convenience and whenever they have questions. Without written instructions, patients may choose to hear what they want to hear. Do you remember the old joke about the ninety-year-old man who was seen by his physician for a physical exam? Three days later, the physician saw the man on the street with a thirty-year-old woman on his arm and a smile on his face. "Thanks, Doc, I did just what you told me, and I've never felt better," said the patient.

"What was that?" asked the physician.

"You told me to find a hot mama and be cheerful," replied the man.

"No," said the physician. "I said, you have a heart murmur and be careful."

Consider Ongoing Support Mechanisms

Be sure to note the risks of failing to follow through on the discharge instructions you give to patients. This is an important part of the informed consent process. It is crucial to provide the prognosis if the patient chooses to ignore the treatment plan.

Help patients by scheduling tests or treatments before they leave the office. Follow-up in ambulatory care settings is more likely when the follow-up or referral appointment is scheduled before the patient leaves the health care setting.

Telephone reminders, whether supplied by you, a member of your staff, a family member, or other groups, can be very effective. Some communities have volunteer services that will call patients to ask whether they have taken their medication. Support groups, whether community, telephone, or Internet based, can provide the ongoing source of motivation needed by some patients.

Be familiar with community support systems and resources. Self-care programs can also increase a patient's confidence in his ability to manage his condition.

Take advantage of public health campaigns that encourage healthy behaviors. Obtain posters for your office, distribute campaign brochures to patients, and offer to participate in screenings and educational offerings. When your patient sees the same poster in your office and on his bus to work each day, he is more likely to believe the message.

Observe for Better Information

Will Rogers said that "people learn more from observation than conversation." You will learn more whenever you can take the time to watch your patient demonstrate recommended techniques. You may have the best models or illustrations, and you may teach in a clear and understandable way, but until you see your patient master what you have taught, you should not feel comfortable that he will achieve the desired results. Success creates self-confidence. Patients who are confident in their ability to follow through are more likely to do just that. Your encouragement is also a form of support, for it conveys respect and helps build confidence and hope. The Swedish physician Alex Munthe (1929), when asked the secret of medical success, replied, "To inspire confidence. The doctor who possesses this gift can practically raise the dead."

Set the Example

Being an example for patients encourages them to follow through. A survey of 1,400 gastroenterologists found that only 35 percent of them adhered to American Cancer Society prevention guidelines for rectal exams, occult blood testing, and sigmoidoscopy. The most common reason given for not following the guidelines was lack of time (Montague, 1995a).

Your expectations should be stated honestly and in a straightforward manner so that your patient understands them. If your expectations differ significantly from those of your patient, you will want to continue the discussion further.

Recognize that when side effects affect your patient's quality of life, the patient is likely to compromise or abandon his treatment regimens. To the patient, future health benefits may not outweigh immediate inconvenience or side effects. Be sure that your patient knows what to expect and has had the opportunity to consider alternatives before choosing treatment.

At the end of every visit, be clear about what you will do and what the patient is going to do before the next visit.

Patients will follow advice only when they trust your competence and believe that you have only their best interest in mind. Most patients are fascinated by what you have to say about them and far less interested in what you have to say about yourself. Patients do things for their own reasons, not yours. What works for one patient may work for another, but not all others. Talk about how follow-through will benefit your patient specifically. For example, "If you lose twenty pounds, we'll be able to give you the medication in liquid form rather than by injection."

Consider Values and Beliefs

Consider your patient's values and beliefs. What he values will be his motivation. In his book *Managing at the Speed of Change*, Daryl R. Conner (1992, p. 164) wrote, "Beliefs are the set of integrated values and expectations that provide a framework for shaping what people hold to be true or false, relevant or irrelevant, good or bad, about their environment." Patients' beliefs are a good predictor of their ability to comply with your treatment plan. Asking if the patient cares about health, agrees with the diagnosis, perceives the condition as serious, feels the recommended treatment will work, fears regimen side effects, or believes the regimen will be difficult to follow, has been recommended to monitor patients' health beliefs (Eracker, Kirscht, and Becker, 1984). What do you need to know and what does the patient need to know in order to have a treatment plan that is rational for both of you?

Involve Family

With your patient's permission, involve his family for support. William Jenner said, "Never believe what a patient tells you his doctor said." Patients who aren't inclined to follow your advice may have a different story to tell their families. With your patient's permission, take time to involve his spouse or others close to him in routine appointments or preoperative visits. Involving others can result in better follow-through and, in the event of an adverse clinical outcome, will have permitted you to develop the rapport with the family that might avert a lawsuit.

Motivate

If the patient needs to make behavioral changes, keep in mind what motivates changes in behavior: money, fear, recognition, and support. Some employers and managed care companies provide better benefits or require lower employee contributions if the patient adheres to an exercise or treatment regimen, for example.

If your patient doesn't follow through due to the cost of your recommended treatment, explain that the treatment is less expensive than hospitalization or the treatment that will be necessary if the illness advances. Case managers can be a wonderful resource for you and your patient when the ability to pay for treatment is an issue.

Simply checking with patients about their follow-through will tend to increase it. Ask your patient to keep a compliance log. Develop a cue system for follow-through and documentation. For example, if an adolescent patient should take his medication twice a day, you might agree that before and after school is the best time. Other patients might choose to keep their medication next to their car keys. If a patient's exercise regimen is to use a treadmill, his cue might be the beginning or end of a television show he watches each day.

CD-ROM technology is becoming more popular as a patient education tool and can encourage follow-through as well. Software can be used to show patients what kind of improvements they can expect if they take their medication as ordered and what the consequences are likely to be if they don't. Some companies that provide pharmacy benefits are beginning to track unfilled prescriptions and alert patients when refills are due.

Responding to Failure to Follow Through

When you detect or the patient admits to a failure to follow through, express concern for the patient first, then warn him of the likely result of his decision not to follow the agreed-upon treatment plan. When a patient tells you that he has not followed the treatment plan, ask open-ended questions such as, "Why do you think that is?" or, "What can you do differently in the future?" Asking closed-ended questions, such as, "Do you agree with this treatment plan?" or, "Will you be able to schedule the blood test today?" may give you the answer you want to hear but fail to alert you to a misunderstanding between you and your patient. Open-ended questions often begin with *what, why, how,* or *tell me.* Close-ended questions often begin with *do, when,* or *which.*

If a patient returns with the same, unimproved symptoms, ask him to describe the treatment he has been following before you consider switching regimens. Merely asking, "Have you taken the medicine as directed?" is a closed-ended question to which the patient may, out of embarrassment or fear, answer yes. Instead, ask, "Let's review what's been happening with you and your condition since your last visit."

When you are speaking with a patient who has not followed through, try not to use the word *but.* It puts your patient on the defensive. Instead, substitute the word *and.* For example, instead of saying, "I know that you are trying to modify your eating, but it's not enough just to cut back; you need to substitute fruits for some of the refined products," try, "I know that you are trying to modify your eating, and it's not just enough to cut back; you need to substitute fruits for some of your candy and baked goods."

Information is a form of support that can change behavior. Most Americans claim that they floss their teeth "almost" every day. What changed one patient's behavior and convinced him to floss daily was his dentist's telling him, "Plaque forms in twenty-four hours. If you don't remove it within twenty-four hours, we have to scrape or chip it off when you come in for a cleaning."

Ask your patient, "If you were the only person in the world who could solve this problem, what would you do?" He may present you with an acceptable plan and will be more likely to comply with it because he feels a sense of ownership of the idea. Treatment plans should be realistic from the patient's point of view whenever possible. Praise the patient for his decision and express confidence in his ability to follow through with his plan. In one study, patients were more satisfied and had higher rates of compliance when they assertively participated in the clinical conversation (Cecil and Killeen, 1997).

Patients with chronic conditions or who need behavior modification can benefit from understanding how habits are developed. In *Empires of the Mind,* Waitley (1995, p. 205) observes, "Habits are formed after the body responds the same way twenty-five or thirty times to identical stimuli. But here's an interesting discovery: After a certain amount of this repetition, the message from the sensory nerves jumps directly to the conditioned motor nerves without a conscious decision by the brain. So while a mere twenty-five or thirty repeats can form a new habit . . . the same number is involved in developing good habits, depending on practice input and supporting environment."

Documenting Failure to Follow Through

Document a patient's postponing or failing to keep an appointment. If you keep your appointment books in pencil and erase names when appointments are canceled or postponed, make a note in the patient's chart. If your situation warrants it, consider an "appointment not kept" stamp that can be stamped into the record. When a patient fails to keep an appointment, his primary caregiver should be asked to determine whether the patient should be contacted by telephone call or with a no-show letter. Prompting the patient with a reminder call or letter prior to his scheduled visit can encourage him to keep the appointment.

Some physicians will threaten termination of the physician-patient relationship as a "last resort." If you are considering terminating your relationship with a patient because of his failure to follow through, be sure that you have specified your expectations about the patient's responsibilities to follow through on the agreed-upon treatment plan. If a mutually acceptable treatment plan cannot be worked out, the patient may do better with another physician.

When a patient has a poor outcome, even if it is the result of his lack of follow-through, he may elect to sue the physician. If the patient files a malpractice suit, he will conveniently forget his failure to follow through with the treatment plan. Patient noncompliance is a frequent defense in malpractice cases. Attorneys are fond of saying, "Noncompliance is always the defense, but is it documented?" In some states, if a patient contributes to his own injury, the percentage of his "contribution" is deducted from a malpractice award. Some physicians fail to document a patient's failure to follow through because it takes time, or they are sure they won't forget, or they consider the risks to be minimal. But documentation serves as a critical reminder to address the issue again when you next see the patient. Document your interventions. Don't be noncompliant about noncompliance.

15

Adverse Patient Outcomes

An injury is much sooner forgotten than an insult.

Philip Chesterfield

One of the most difficult challenges a physician faces is handling an adverse patient outcome. Knowing that patients can and often do associate an unexpected adverse outcome with negligence, a physician may try to say as little as possible, hoping that the situation will resolve itself. Or she may act defensively, trying to explain what happened in terms of how the patient might have contributed to the situation.

When an unexpected adverse outcome occurs and there may be significant out-of-pocket expenses for the patient, the health care team and the patient must maintain excellent relationships if a lawsuit is to be prevented. Anticipating that adverse outcomes will occur and being aware of strategies for handling these situations both before and after they occur are important tools in managing patient expectations.

Advance Handling

In the early stages of illness, your patient probably knows more about his condition than you do. Listen to your patient in order to have the best possible information.

The consent discussion is your best opportunity to detect unrealistic expectations. Don't protect your patient from the expected disease course. Don't guarantee results. In the long run, you may be doing the patient a disservice and damaging your reputation in the process. Explain that complications, such as infections, can and do occur. Patients should be authorizing, rather than merely agreeing to, the procedure or treatment plan. The patient who has assumed responsibility for a decision is less likely to blame you if the outcome is less than he hoped for.

Advising patients about what they can expect, even for very routine matters, is important. Many malpractice claims involve bad results that take patients by surprise. In a study of communication styles of primary care physicians (Levinson and others, 1997), physicians who had no malpractice claim history were more likely to orient patients about what was going to happen next: "First, I'm going to examine you, and then we will talk the problem over." Physicians in this group were also more likely to ask patients for their opinions, use humor, and spend a few more minutes with their patients.

Make it a standard operating procedure to advise patients to call if their problem worsens or if they feel dissatisfied with their progress. If you say to a patient, "Call me in a week," the patient may experience an untoward event on the fourth day but wait to call you. Instead say, "Call me in a week, or sooner if you aren't satisfied with your progress." Make sure that your patient knows how to reach you.

Watch for the Red Flag

Recognize that a red flag is waving whenever a patient returns with the same acute problem. Do not allow your earlier assumptions to govern your thoughts and actions. Listen as though you were hearing the patient's story for the first time. Learn from the tragic experiences of others. Whenever a catastrophic event occurs in medicine, one of these two questions is often raised: "Why didn't someone just ask the patient?" or, "Why didn't we just listen to the patient?" When patients give you a warning, take it. Eric Anderson (1996, p. 15) wrote of his experience as a physician caring for a patient who would later sue him for malpractice: "I said 'in my opinion.' We tend to forget that patients have opinions too. We don't always ask for them." Encourage patients to speak up whenever they have a question or something doesn't seem right. The patient who feels comfortable questioning why a medication looks different or why the technician is preparing to draw blood from the "wrong" arm is helping you prevent a possible adverse event.

Mistakes happen when someone knows something but fails to tell someone else. In a study of adverse outcomes involving children (Pichert and others, 1997), researchers found that 35 percent of the outcomes were attributable to communication failures among health professionals or between them and their patients. Set up systems, such as having everyone review the logs of calls taken during off hours, as a way to improve communication with everyone in your practice.

Aftermath

Take care of the patient's medical needs first and keep those needs as the focus of *all* of your discussions. The patient's needs must be at the center of every message.

Although it is prudent to notify your professional liability carrier as quickly as possible, do not avoid the patient and family. A delay in communicating bad news to a patient can place nurses in a difficult position in their relationships with the patient or family (Miranda and Brody, 1992). If you don't know why a situation has occurred, talk with your patient about what has happened and what the next steps will be. For example, say something like, "I don't have all of the answers yet. Let's see what the

> Take care of the patient's medical needs first and keep those needs as the focus of *all* of your discussions.

test results [or specialists] tell us." If you put off the patient or family, they will fill in any gaps with interpretations from their well-meaning but certainly less-knowledgeable friends or acquaintances. Understand that the patient and the family may need to hear your message several times before they really hear it. A hospital risk manager has said that "working with the family after an adverse event is like wrestling with a gorilla. You rest when the gorilla wants to rest." Do not minimize the patient's and family's concerns. Keep your language free of jargon. Encourage questions so that you can assess understanding of the situation. If appropriate, use "we" to show empathy.

When preparing for the first meeting with the patient or family, keep several thoughts in mind:

• Analyze the situation from the patient's and family's points of view only. Develop the points that you want the patient to understand. Anticipate the kinds of perceptions and responses he could have that are very different from yours. What is your answer to each of those perceptions and responses? Why should the patient believe you?

• If there are several physicians or organizations involved, consider having one spokesperson for the health care team and one for the family. The spokespersons must be committed to frequent communications between them and their constituents. Others who are questioned can make notes of the questions and refer to the spokesperson. "That's a good question. Let's write it down so that we can remember to ask Dr. Gray about it."

• Understand that your patient will want to know why the adverse event or outcome occurred. In preparation for your meeting, ask and respond to the question "Why?" five times after each statement you plan to make to the patient.

• Prepare to meet with the patient, the family, or both in a quiet, uninterrupted setting (no phones, no beepers). "What will be said is often among the most important communications the patient or family have ever heard and they can feel slighted and uncared for if the physician is allowed to be distracted during this time. People find it comforting to receive their physicians' full attention and concern" (Miranda and Brody, 1992, p. 83).

Begin your meeting by preparing the patient and family: "I'm afraid I have some information that isn't good." A cartoon showed a surgeon leaving the OR and saying to the patient's spouse, "Is your husband a good sport?" Of course, from the family's perspective, the problem with being a good sport is that you have to lose to be one.

Crisis mismanagement is taking a bad situation and making it worse. Don't use the telephone to give bad news if it is at all possible to meet with the patient and family in person. Insensitivity in giving bad news will be remembered. One patient referred to a telephone call from his physician as the "death notice by telephone." The family of another patient was incensed that the physician chose to speak to them by telephone—from another floor in the hospital.

When practical, allow the patient to get dressed before giving bad news and speak with no physical barriers between you. Listen to determine how much the patient knows and how much he wants to know (Michaels, 1992).

Keep the patient's needs as the sole focus of every discussion you have. Avoid becoming defensive or making excuses. Don't malign the patient or family, even if you can. Don't criticize or ask questions that imply criticism of the patient or family. It will seem self-serving to ask, "Were you giving your mother the medications I prescribed according to schedule?" Instead ask, "Let's review the medications your mom was taking to see if there might be some explanation there."

If the patient requires transfer to an intensive care unit, the needs of the family may shift somewhat. A study of family members of ICU patients (Foss and Tenholder, 1993) found that they wanted staff to give directions about what to do at the bedside, to receive more support from their own families, to have a place to be alone as a family unit in the hospital, to be informed in advance of plans to transfer the patient, and to have flexibility in the time allowed for visiting the patient. When your patient is very sick, don't focus so intently on his physical condition that you forget to use your rapport-building skills with the patient (if possible) and with the family.

Keep the patient or family informed of what the next steps will be and when they will occur. This will return some control to your patient and will help him prepare for the future. If the patient or family member is having difficulty responding to you, ask, "What are you feeling?" and empathize with that emotion.

Don't Abandon the Patient

Follow through on whatever you say you will do. One study (Beckman, Markakis, Suchman, and Frankel, 1994) revealed that the decision to litigate often followed a perceived failure on the part of the physician to stay connected with the patient. Plaintiffs described unsuccessful attempts to reach the physician through the answering service, unkept promises to return to the bedside, telephone calls that were not returned, and delegation of care to residents or junior members of the team. Harvard Medical School psychiatrist Harold J. Bursztajn believes that if a patient feels abandoned, one way for him to continue the relationship is to file a lawsuit. Patients who have received follow-up attention are less likely to sue than those who don't, Bursztajn maintains (1997).

In one malpractice case, the plaintiff sued the hospital and one of its nurses after an unexpected incident. While being placed on a bedpan, the patient heard a crack and said to the nurse, "I think you just broke my leg." The nurse dismissed the comment and did not report it or take any action. Hours later, the patient told a physician, who ordered radiographs. There was a fracture, and the patient was transferred to an orthopedic unit. The nurse did not visit the patient. The plaintiff said that she knew that the nurse would not be liable for any damages because the nurse was insured by the hospital, but that she wanted to teach the nurse a lesson.

In a study of forty-five plaintiff depositions (Beckman, Markakis, Suchman, and Frankel, 1994), 71 percent of the plaintiffs discussed the problems they experienced in the physician-patient relationship. When asked why they sued, they most frequently cited feeling abandoned by the physician. Plaintiffs also cited their physician's devaluing the views of the patient or family, delivering information poorly, and failing to understand the patient's or family's perspective.

Help the patient or family identify helpful resources, such as social workers, support groups, or pastoral care associates, but don't let them feel that you are transferring them completely to those resources.

Use empathy and compassion to keep the relationship with your patient as positive as possible during what will be a stressful time for both of you. Give assurance of your ongoing relationship. If your relationship is changing because a specialist is assuming primary responsibility for the patient, provide detailed information about how you will stay involved. For example: "Yes, I will still be your medical doctor. We will see each other as often as needed, starting with our next appointment in two weeks" or, "Yes, I will still be your doctor. Dr. Gomez will be performing surgery, and I will be in to see you afterwards, and you can call me anytime you have questions. When Dr. Gomez feels that you're ready, he'll refer you back to me."

"I'll be with you every step of the way" is a powerfully comforting message.

When a Mistake Has Been Made

Witman, Park, and Hardin (1996) conducted a study to examine patients' attitudes toward physician error. They surveyed patients of an outpatient clinic of a university medical center about three scenarios, involving a minor mistake, a moderate mistake, and a severe mistake. For each scenario the researchers asked patients the same questions about how they would prefer the physician to communicate after the mistake. Almost all of the patients reported that they wanted their physician to disclose the mistake, even if it was minor. Physicians may fear that in disclosing a mistake they will have to apologize for it and that the apology will be interpreted as an admission of liability. Apologizing for an adverse outcome should be considered on a case-by-case basis. You may receive conflicting advice. Some experts may suggest that you "tell the truth and tell it fast," whereas other advisers may suggest that you "tell them as little as possible as slowly as possible." Your credibility as a physician is more important than your legal positioning. Bursztajn and Brodsky (1996, p. 2061) suggest that a statement such as, "I made a mistake here; I did my best to remedy it," can eliminate a patient's need to go to court to force an acknowledgment of the error.

When a mistake has caused injury, patients and families are often heard to say that they want to be sure that the same mistake won't injure another patient. Let your patient and your staff know about action you are taking to prevent the mistake from happening again in the future. Assurance that a lesson has been learned may prevent patients, families, or staff from leaking information to the press in order to force action.

If the press inquires, cite patient confidentiality as your reason not to discuss the case, unless you have the patient's written permission to speak about the situation. And then be conservative. Stick to the facts without blaming anyone. Of course, it's helpful to be able to say something like, "The patient was in a life-threatening situation, and an informed decision was made by his family to proceed with surgery."

When trust has been broken, people often stop talking, and problems remain unresolved. It may be up to you to keep the channels of communication open. People are more likely to remember the first and last things you say to them. End your meeting with a reference to your next meeting or with the option of a future meeting.

Unexpected Death of a Patient

When death is unexpected, the patient's family does not have time to prepare. It may be necessary to give information in small quantities, so let family members know that you are available for another meeting or whenever questions arise. A surgeon in Greenwich, Connecticut, tells family members of a patient who dies, whether the death was expected or unexpected, "You may have more questions tomorrow or even next year. If questions come up, please call me. I will be happy to answer them or meet with you at any time."

Many people need assistance coping with major unexpected change. Airlines have learned that having trained grief counselors to help families after a plane crash is greatly appreciated. Their crisis teams are therefore always at the ready. In one study of bereaved parents (Harper and Wisian, 1994), parents' satisfaction with their physician was linked to the physician's being available, providing medical information, and providing grief counseling. The same study found that these three satisfiers were less likely to be offered when the parents were reassigned to another physician after their child's death.

Physicians and staff often ask about appropriate expressions of condolences. In our culture, a condolence visit by any member of the health care team is remarkable and highly valued. A visit to the family's observance does not take very long and is actually more thoughtful than flowers. The family will treasure a sincere note of condolence mentioning a memory of the patient. Paul R. Keane, a Boston attorney, cautions that "a sympathy card is appropriate— just don't include your final bill with it" (Paul R. Keane, personal communication to the author, 1996).

Be conscientious about reviewing the bills of patients who have experienced unexpected adverse outcomes. When a patient has lost income or incurred additional expenses, your attempts to collect monies due may be perceived as adding insult to injury. Your state may have a provision that failing to bill a patient or writing off a bill cannot be used as evidence of liability in a malpractice case. Some attorneys advise sending one bill and then "forgetting" to send any more.

• • • • • • •

In summary, anticipate that unexpected adverse outcomes will occur, and manage expectations accordingly. Do not blame the patient or family. Try to minimize any out-of-pocket expenses that the patient or family will have as a result of the adverse event or outcome. Keep your patient informed about what will happen next and assure him of your continuing availability and support.

16

. . . .

When Patients Leave

A bad attitude will only seal a closed door.

Linda Richardson

If you walked into your office tomorrow and discovered that a $3,000 computer was missing, how much time and effort would you devote to finding out how that loss occurred? Well, you have patients worth ten and a hundred times that who are walking out your door forever. How much time and effort are you devoting to those losses? There is no need to guess why patients left, when you can ask them. Former patients possess valuable information about flaws in your practice and the appeal of your competitors. Yet many physicians and practice managers feel uncomfortable asking former patients about their decision to leave the practice. Why is it that some practices will chase a patient to the ends of the earth for a $50 balance due but are afraid to contact former patients who have decided to seek care elsewhere? Although it may be too late to fix a situation for a patient who has left, the information you receive may motivate you to take focused action to make improvements for your practice.

When dissatisfied patients leave your practice, a bad public image can result. If your patient has to explain to a managed care organization why he is leaving, you may be asked to respond to the patient's claims. Health plans themselves are being graded on disenrollments. Although disenrollments might not be a reliable gauge of quality, they are viewed by many analysts as a very objective measure of member satisfaction.

Patients, even those in restricted managed care networks, do not want to be treated as though they have no other options, because they do. Sam Walton (1993) said it best: "There is only one boss: the customer. And he can fire everybody in the company from the Chairman on down, simply by spending his dollars somewhere else."

Inactive Patients

The first step in surveying former patients is to determine who is no longer using your services and why. Differentiate between lost patients and inactive patients. Don't automatically assume that a patient who has requested a copy of his medical record is seeking care elsewhere. The patient may be inactive, not lost. Inactive patients should be contacted on a routine basis. Review the patient's medical record prior to the call and structure the call around the patient's welfare. The objective of the call should not be to book an appointment for the patient. A patient who feels pressured to make an appointment may agree to it but not keep it.

Some organizations excel at regular follow-up with inactive customers. At the Adam Broderick Image Group in Ridgefield, Connecticut, clients receive the "How are you?" letter shown in Exhibit 16.1 three months after their last visit to the salon. Another letter (Exhibit 16.2) reassures clients that they are welcome even if they have tried another salon.

At-Risk Patients

At any given time, you have patients in your practice who are at risk to leave you for another physician. Certainly, those patients

Exhibit 16.1. "How Are You?" Letter.

Dear Mrs. Malloy:

We are sorry that you have not returned since your March 16 appointment. We don't want to lose you! You are a valued client and we want to continue to be your salon. To ensure the same care you have come to expect, we have retained a history of your records as well as the products you have purchased at the salon.

The staff joins me in extending a special invitation to you to come in at your earliest convenience. I look forward to reviewing with you the exceptional qualifications of our personnel. The few minutes spent matching your requirements with their skills will guarantee that you will continue to receive the specific services you want from the people you trust and like. We'll work very hard to please you. Come see us soon!

Please give me a call; I'd love to hear from you!

Very truly yours,

Adam

Source: Adam Broderick Image Group. Used with permission.

who indicate on surveys that they would not recommend you are at high risk to defect. At the Williamsport Hospital in Williamsport, Pennsylvania, a corporate officer personally visits the home of any patient who indicates on a patient satisfaction survey that he will not return in the future. Assessing patient satisfaction and responding to unmet expectations is critical to retention of patients. Have a mechanism for staff members to alert you whenever a patient is angry or upset.

Some department stores station staff members at the exits to ask customers leaving without a purchase what they came for that they didn't find. It's an opportunity to correct any misconceptions the customer may have or to gain information about customers' unmet

Exhibit 16.2. "Welcome Back" Letter.

Dear Ms. Dwyer:

It has been over three months since your visit on November 23 and we're sorry that we haven't seen you since then.

If there is a special concern about some aspect of your experience here, I'd very much like to hear from you. Your comments and opinions are important to me—and to everyone on the staff. If you have decided to try the services of another spa or salon, please rest assured that you are still welcome here. Just let us know what we can do to meet your needs.

As a valued client, your satisfaction is of the utmost importance to us. We have retained complete historical and lab records of all the specific spa and salon services you have received at the Adam Broderick Image Group. We firmly believe that paying attention to the details is key to building a lasting, successful relationship.

I do hope you will accept this invitation to visit us again soon. Please don't hesitate to call with any questions or comments.

Very truly yours,

Adam

Source: Adam Broderick Image Group. Used with permission.

---

needs. The president of one manufacturer of laptop computers personally calls potential customers who contact his company but buy elsewhere.

Some patients will be at risk to leave when they change employers. A patient may believe that he is required to choose a physician listed in a directory given to him by his new employer. Perhaps he is unaware of an available out-of-network option. Perhaps you participate with the new managed care company, but the directory is inaccurate or you have elected not to have your name listed because you aren't accepting new patients. Stay in touch with patients who tell you that they are looking to change jobs. When you see a newspaper notice that a patient of yours has taken a new job, call the patient to congratulate him. It will give him an opportunity to talk about any problems concerning insurance coverage.

How well would your physicians and staff handle a request from a patient to change from one physician to another in your practice? Women have long encountered this situation when they want to try a different stylist in their hair salon but leave the salon rather than risk upsetting their present stylist. Let staff know that requests to change physicians within the practice should be handled graciously, with no questions asked. "Of course" should be the response to such a request.

One practice was stunned to receive a note from a patient asking for her records to be transferred to another physician. The practice manager telephoned her and learned that the patient didn't want to be treated in one of their exam rooms. She had received bad news in that room. The practice manager assured the patient that she understood how she felt and would be more than happy to respect her needs. The patient happily continued with the practice as a result of the practice manager's willingness to contact her and honor her preference.

Surveying Former Patients

Contacting former associates, whether they are employees, patients, or customers, can have multiple benefits. For example, exit interviews of customers can result in sales. One credit card service organization found that a telephone call to question cardholders who had stopped using their cards led to the immediate reinstatement of one-third of the defectors (Heskett and others, 1994).

Frederick F. Reichheld, author of The Loyalty Effect (1996), advises companies with declining market shares to require senior executives to telephone former customers. Those executives should ask "Why?" five times to reach the root cause of the customer's reason for defection. Telephoning former customers is not anyone's favorite thing to do, Reichheld admits. "Most people don't relish the idea of phoning strangers, let alone strangers who've been unhappy with the value they've received, and you will have to overcome that reluctance with leadership, peer pressure, and if necessary, a chair and whip. There is simply no substitute for having senior executives learn directly from defectors why the company's value proposition is inadequate" (p. 213).

The following is an example of how root cause analysis could work:

QUESTION: Why did you leave XYZ Medical Associates?
ANSWER: Well, I guess I just didn't feel comfortable there anymore.
QUESTION: Why didn't you feel comfortable there anymore?
ANSWER: Well, the practice merged with another practice and things became very different.
QUESTION: How were things different?
ANSWER: They got very pushy.
QUESTION: How did they get pushy?
ANSWER: Well, they wanted to be paid even before you saw the doctor. You can check my records. I always paid my bills, but suddenly I was being treated like a deadbeat.
QUESTION: What made you feel that way?
ANSWER: It was the way they said things. For instance, you'd give your name, and the very next thing they would say was, "Do you want to pay by check or credit card?"

Training to help employees build rapport before requesting payment would help this practice prevent future patient defections.

Another way to approach former patients is to call them and ask, "To help us better serve our patients in the future, what were the factors that led you to select a new physician?" You will find out whether other practices are providing better service or whether there is a perception issue. It is easy to assume that you know why patients leave, but the answers they give may not be the ones you thought were most important.

Mail Survey of Former Patients

For those who can't be persuaded by the leadership, peer pressure, or chair and whip suggested by Reichheld, a mail survey can still uncover useful information. One practice's survey of former patients is shown in Exhibit 16.3.

Consider hosting a focus group of former patients. You might find out that something happened to make working with your practice less convenient. One physician was surprised to hear how strongly patients felt about having to file their own insurance forms

Exhibit 16.3. Mail Survey of Former Patients.

1. Our records indicate that you are no longer obtaining care at [name of organization]. Is that correct?

2. What is the main reason that led you to seek medical care elsewhere? Any other reasons?

3. Did anyone help you decide to seek care elsewhere? Who?

4. Please think back to your original decision to seek care at [name of organization]. What led you initially to seek care there?

5. Overall, would you say that [name of organization] exceeded, met, or fell below your expectations? How?

6. Are you currently receiving medical care elsewhere?

7. Where and why?

8. What led you to select [name of new provider]?

9. What, if anything, could have been done to keep you as a patient?

Thank you for your comments. Your answers will help us to better serve our patients.

after the practice stopped providing that service. Other feedback might be that costs were higher than expected or that office hours were perceived as inconvenient or inadequate. If you identify misconceptions, you should communicate correct information to all patients in the practice, so that at-risk patients don't defect for the same reason(s). For example, one patient explained that she no longer needed to see a gynecologist because she was in menopause. The practice increased its patient education materials on menopause.

Focus groups can convey important information to you about the new practices patients have selected. The facilitator might ask, "Why do you like your new practice better than being cared for by XYZ Medical Associates?" The follow-up question would then be, "Why are those factors important to you?"

We Want You Back

Some patients may have left your practice because they thought they would save money, or their spouses talked them into changing, or they weren't really dissatisfied but just felt like trying someone new. These patients might be embarrassed to return to your practice, particularly if they had copies of their medical records sent to another physician. They might be afraid that someone will question them or say, "We could have told you so." Knowing that they would be welcomed back to the practice would make a big difference to patients who would like to return. Whenever you send a copy of the patient's medical record to another organization, send a note to the patient letting him know that you have done so and express interest in his health. Even if the patient doesn't return, this kind of thoughtfulness can generate positive word of mouth for your practice. One practice sent the results of a pap smear to a patient who had transferred to another practice. The nurse wrote on the bottom of the report, "Good luck with your upcoming surgery." The patient talked about this gesture to dozens of friends.

Another way to encourage patients to return to your practice is to keep former patients on your mailing list for at least five years. A personal note jotted on your direct mail piece, such as, "Hope all is well with you," lets the former patient know that he isn't receiving information simply because you haven't updated your mailing list. Send former patients announcements of new personnel, extended office hours, and new health plan affiliations. Even if a patient doesn't elect to return to your practice, this is an excellent strategy to improve the perceptions of former patients about your practice.

When DDB Needham, an advertising agency, lost the McDonald's account, the CEO was determined to win it back. He provided unsolicited ad campaigns, strategic advice, promotional reports, and research papers. He became a board member for a Ronald McDonald House, the chain's charity. He maintained a readiness to do business with McDonald's again, should the company choose. It took sixteen years, but ultimately McDonald's did return to DDB Needham (Beatty, 1997).

At my college, members of the senior class had the privilege of voting for the commencement speaker. One year, columnist Art Buchwald lost out in the election to Father Daniel Berrigan. The following year, Buchwald sent a letter to the students, letting them know that he held no grudge. He reminded the students of his charm and sex appeal and enclosed a "Honk If You Still Love Nixon" bumper sticker. Buchwald was elected by a tremendous margin to speak at the next commencement.

◆　◆　◆　◆　◆　◆　◆

Lesson learned: don't be bitter or look to blame others for a failed relationship. Learn what you can and use the experience to improve your relationship with other patients. Maintain a sense of humor and find ways to let former patients know that you would welcome their return.

> **Don't be bitter or look to blame others for a failed relationship.**

Part V

· ·

Exceeding Expectations

17

Respecting Patient Preferences

The more you remember about a person, the more deeply you compliment that person.

Harry Lorayne

Patients value experiences in which their unique preferences are identified and respected. That's why remembering that your patient prefers capsules to tablets or likes a certain exam room can make a routine office visit special. Respecting preferences is a proven strategy in meeting and exceeding patient expectations.

Know Your Patient

A classic customer service story about the importance of knowing customers involves General Motors. GM introduced one of its cars, the Chevy Nova, into its Spanish-speaking markets before finding out that in Spanish, *no va* means "no go."

Respecting preferences requires personal knowledge of your patient and his needs. Know what's important to your patient. If you are not sure, ask about or observe how your patient spends his discretionary time and money. What people spend their extra time and money on is what matters to them, and you can use those subjects to make quick connections with patients.

The more you know about your patient, the easier it is to help him decide on what he needs. Companies that focus on building relationships quickly become skilled at giving customers more than they expect. This can only happen when a customer's preferences are known. In medicine, you can use your knowledge of the patient and what the expected disease course will be to anticipate and respond to patient needs.

Understand Your Patient's Values

What are your patient's values? Achieving goals? Having power? Being a respected member of society? Making the world a better place? Having fun and enjoying life? Living traditionally? Being able to work? Being able to interact with other people? Being able to sleep through the night? Does your patient prefer a physician-patient relationship that is collegial and friendly or one in which the physician is more authoritative?

Listen to how patients frame their relationships with you. The patient who says, "Do you remember the time you came in during the snowstorm to see me?" values the longevity of your association. If you take the time to recall experiences that you have shared, you will be connecting with the patient in a meaningful way.

Recognize Special Events and Interests

Recognize significant events in your patient's life. Everyone appreciates receiving an extra clipping of a birth or wedding announcement, promotion, or award. This effort does not have to be cumbersome. Jot a one-line note on your business card, clip it to the news item, and mail. You will be amazed at the response you will receive to this thoughtful gesture. When I spoke about this strategy with a class of physician assistants, one student recalled the joy she felt when her dentist sent her a clipping about her graduation from college with a congratulatory note. When you take time to acknowledge the special events in a patient's life, you are saying that you are interested in your patient as a person.

You don't have to wait for a significant event. Sending a news clipping about a subject of interest to your patient is just as effective. For example, if your patient mentions that he likes to vacation in Portugal, you could send him an article on that country. A patient who is starting a business would welcome any information about that subject. It won't matter if he has seen the article or if he already knows all the information contained in it. It's the thought that counts. If you don't have time to send mail, file articles of interest with the patient's record and give them to him during the next visit.

Honor Patient Preferences

Remembering and respecting needs is a proven strategy for creating loyal relationships. At Ritz Carlton hotels, for example, the usual brand of soft drinks stocked in the hotel room mini-bars will be replaced throughout the hotel if a competing soft drink company is hosting a conference there. Once a person has stayed at a Ritz Carlton and indicated her preferences, she can be sure that in future stays she will be given a nonsmoking room, on an upper floor, with detachable clothes hangers in the closet (or whatever it was she specified). It's the hotel's way of saying, "We appreciate your business." Ritz Carlton advertises this respect for customer preferences in their ads, which read, "Why settle for a hotel that just remembers your name when you can stay at a hotel that remembers your needs?" (Schneiderman, 1996).

Consultants may refer to this strategy as database marketing or segment-of-one marketing. Whatever name you give to it, it's a system for remembering information about your patient that shows you really care. For some people, the system that's inside their head is all they need. Others keep notes on Rolodex cards, in the "Other" section of medical records, or in a database management program such as ACT or Telemagic. Whatever system you use, you will make an impact. Wally Lamb, author of *She's Come Undone*, told the *New*

York Times a story of his relationship with Oprah Winfrey. "Oprah had called me back in 1992 when the book first came out, just as a fan, to say how much she liked it. I was doing laundry at the time and almost fell into the spin cycle. This time when she called in January [1997] she asked, 'Are you still doing the laundry?'" What was remarkable was that Oprah Winfrey had remembered something personal "about" him (Fitzpatrick, 1997).

Establish a System for Recording Preferences

What patients want and expect may seem simple to them, but responding to these requests can present a challenge for your practice. Keeping notes on patient preferences increases your chances of remembering them in the future. A master problem log gives you, at a glance, a quick review of past problems. Patients love it when you ask, "How's the knee?" and the knee was a problem years before. With information recorded, you are more likely to recall that the patient prefers early morning appointments and that she asks for mammograms frequently because her college roommate died of breast cancer at age thirty-two. Take a moment to jot down the names of your patient's spouse and children too.

Harrah's Entertainment, Inc., has established an extensive database of information on customers who visit its casinos. Harrah's records purchases, satisfaction survey responses, and information purchased from credit card companies to learn whether customers are strictly loyal to Harrah's or not. The amassed information is used to determine what customers' preferences are, how much they can be expected to gamble, and what perks they should receive (Binkley, 1997).

Your system doesn't have to be as comprehensive as Harrah's or Oprah's. One physician told me that the most successful patient relations strategy he ever adopted was to record the last thing his patient told him as he was leaving the visit. He would then mention that subject at the beginning of the next visit. It didn't matter what it was; his patients were flattered that he remembered.

A group practice has a section on its patient history form called "What Makes Our Patients Smile." In this section, staff record statements, stories, or other things that have made a patient smile.

Give Choice

Choice is the most cherished American value. People choose their elected officials and just about everything else. Recognizing the value of choice, many managed care companies are now offering employers point-of-service (POS) plans for their employees. Even when employees don't choose the POS plan, they like knowing that they could choose it.

Giving choice helps patients feel that they are receiving just what they want. When you visit a restaurant to have eggs, you expect the server to ask you how you like your eggs cooked. If instead you were brought eggs the way the chef liked to cook them, would you be satisfied? Only if the chef happened to have the same preference for eggs that you did.

Regis McKenna, author of *Real Time: Preparing for the Age of the Never Satisfied Customer* (1997), believes that in order to earn customers' complete approval, leaders have to understand that customers now expect to be asked about their individual preferences and to be treated as if those preferences mattered. Medicine, despite being just about the most intimate profession there is, has been slow to catch on to this. Patients comment that office staff do not recognize them even though they have been patients of the practice for years.

Using your intimate knowledge of a patient's desires, fears, and preferences enables you to meet his expectations and create a loyal relationship. Respecting preferences starts with simply paying attention. How much attention do patients want when they arrive? Everyone wants to be greeted with a smile, but some people then want to read magazines or finish paperwork they have brought with them, whereas others ease their nervousness by making conversation with the receptionist. Allowing patients to make choices reduces anxiety and increases patient satisfaction. You give choice when you ask, "Would you like to have a seat?" instead of saying, "Take a seat." You give choice when you ask: "Would you like a reminder telephone call on the day before your appointment?" "What day is best for your next appointment?" "Please let me know if this becomes too painful and you want me to stop for a moment." "Would you like to wait for the results or should we call you later today?"

Pressure to see more patients in less time often results in limited opportunities for patients to talk about their preferences. In a study of community-acquired pneumonia (Coley and others, 1996), researchers found that more explicit discussion of patient preferences regarding location of care yielded care that was both more highly valued by patients and less costly. Patient preferences for life-sustaining treatments are often based on their values and beliefs. An older patient may value not being a burden to his family, for example. In a study of patient preferences for specific aspects of a cardiac rehabilitation regimen (Moore and Kramer, 1996), researchers found that preferences for convenience (drive time, transportation, noninterference with other life activities, and ease of learning the exercises) were well met, whereas preferences for being able to discuss progress with a professional and choosing one's own exercises were not.

The consent discussion offers a practical opportunity to explore and respect preferences. "I feel that either of these birth control measures will work well for you. Which do you prefer?"

Being flexible and responsive to patient needs means recognizing that there can be more than one right answer to a question. One way to let patients know that they are appreciated is to be flexible when they have special requests. Elizabeth Hilts (1996), a Connecticut restaurant critic, told her readers why New York Ray's was one of her favorite places: "My affection for Ray's stems from the time I called and asked if they could customize one of their specialty pizzas. 'Sure we can,' was the reply. 'This is New York Ray's, where dreams come true.'" When a patient asks you for something, before you automatically say no, consider whether there is a way to accommodate the patient's request. Treating the patient as an individual by respecting his preferences creates the emotional link that strengthens your relationship.

· · · · · · ·

If you know who your patients are, and remember what they want, and are willing to treat different patients differently, you will create very positive and loyal patient relationships.

18

. . . .

Building Loyal Relationships

Wise sayings often fall on barren ground; but a kind
word is never thrown away.

Arthur Helps

There are key strategies for developing and maintaining loyal relationships with your patients. This chapter addresses confidentiality, knowing your patient, using empathy, being a resource, acting consistently, letting your patient know what will happen next, being responsive, and connecting with patients in the office and between visits. The chapter concludes with a model for using ten strategies that can help your practice achieve the balance of consistency and flexibility that is so important in managing patient expectations.

Protect Patient Confidentiality

If you have someone in your life—a friend, relative, clergy member, or physician—with whom you can share any secret, you know how much you value that relationship. Security can be defined as freedom from danger, risk, or doubt. Patients need to feel secure regarding the confidentiality of the information they provide to you. "Will she discuss what I tell her with anyone else?" is an unspoken fear that prevents some patients from providing you with complete and honest information.

There is no faster way to build a foundation of trust than to be absolutely fanatical about patient confidentiality. Letting a patient know that you are committed to protecting patient confidentiality will cement your relationship faster than almost anything else you can do. A qualitative study (Carman and Britten, 1995) explored patients' expectations and attitudes about the confidentiality of their records. The researchers found that expectations were very different than actual experience. Most of the patients felt that administrative and clerical staff should not have access to medical records. They had particular concerns about having nonmedical information in their records and about the confidentiality of computerized records.

And concerned they should be. Mark Hays (1997), chief technology officer and senior vice president of Health+Cast in Philadelphia, says that data systems that depend on simple passwords or key cards can be accessed by high school students. Someone wanting to steal your actual records would have to break in and find the information, but a computer hacker can browse through files, copying some or all of them "while he is sitting at home, 2,000 miles away, eating a pizza" (p. 102). Hays recommends that leaders be proactive about ensuring the security of their information systems.

Three benefits are realized when patients know that you and your organization truly care about their privacy: (1) patients have greater peace of mind, (2) you have the opportunity to differentiate yourself from others providing the same services, and (3) you minimize the risk that outcome studies will be flawed due to inaccurate information provided by patients who are concerned about the confidentiality of their information.

All employees who have access to patient information must understand their obligation to protect that information from unauthorized disclosure. This cannot be overemphasized. If you do not promote this awareness, you may find yourself with employees who rationalize that disclosure is acceptable for some "greater good." Three steps help you create and maintain awareness: developing a strict policy, requiring signed confidentiality agreements, and providing ongoing education and training.

Develop a Patient Confidentiality Policy

You should have a strict policy stating that you do not share even the names of your patients, except as required by law or with a patient's authorization. The statement should emphasize in the strongest possible language that any breach of confidentiality will result in dismissal from your practice or organization. With a strict policy, you and members of your team are less likely to err and release information that you don't consider confidential but that your patient does. Someone working in an orthopedic practice might say, "Well, what's the big deal? Everyone can see that he has his arm in a sling." The big deal is that when you divulge anything about a patient, the patient fears that you might share other, perhaps more confidential information as well. Exhibit 18.1 shows an example of a patient confidentiality policy statement.

Require a Confidentiality Agreement Signed by All Staff Members

Confidentiality agreements are becoming more and more common. Requiring staff members to sign confidentiality agreements on an annual basis is a good way to maintain awareness of the importance of protecting patients' privacy. Exhibit 18.2 shows a sample confidentiality agreement.

Provide Ongoing Confidentiality Education and Training

Most people want to do the right thing, but they don't always know what the right thing is. And for some people, it is not enough to tell them what to do: you also have to tell them why they should do it. Education and training help everyone in the practice maintain sensitivity to the issue of patient confidentiality.

Exhibit 18.1. Policy Statement Regarding Patient Confidentiality.

Our patients must have absolute confidence that all of the information we work with is kept confidential. Please follow these procedures:

Don't share any information, including the names of patients. If you don't reveal the names of patients, you are less likely to err by releasing information that you don't consider confidential but that the patient does.

Do secure information when you are not working with it. Do not leave patient information in unattended areas or where others might see it.

Don't have conversations with or about patients where other people can overhear you.

Do keep in mind what Deborah Norton of Newton-Wellesley Hospital in Massachusetts tells her staff: "Access codes are like toothbrushes. They should be used daily, changed often, and never shared with anyone else."

Don't participate in casual conversations about patients in public places or on the telephone where your conversation might be overheard.

Do call the recipient of any information transmitted by fax and ask that he or she stand by to receive the fax. Then call to be sure he or she has received it.

Don't show the appointment book to patients when booking their appointments.

Do position computer screens so that they don't face the public.

Don't discuss patients with other patients.

Don't post appointment schedules where patients can see them.

Don't put any type of patient information in the trash without destroying it first.

Do ask patients on the intake form whether it is permissible for you to leave messages on their voice mail or answering machine.

Don't show actual patient records when meeting with job applicants or potential consultants or vendors.

Exhibit 18.1. Policy Statement Regarding Patient Confidentiality, cont'd.

Do be conscientious about obtaining the patient's permission before releasing information to family members and employers, that is, people to whom you might assume the patient would want to give information.

Don't use sign-in sheets, especially the kind that ask for the patient's chief complaint. (An alternative is to have numbered pads printed. The patient signs the top sheet, tears it off, and gives it to the receptionist, who uses the information just as the sign-in sheet information is used.)

Do be particularly careful about releasing information to people you might assume have a right to the information, such as other health care providers. Don't permit access to patient information by unauthorized personnel. Health care professionals waiting for the records of their patients should not be permitted to browse through other records.

Breaches of confidentiality can occur in social situations where all of the participants are health care professionals. If you are in doubt, err on the side of the patient and ask your supervisor for advice.

Do be conscientious about preventing access to patient information by members of your family. Unless they are also working in the health care field, you should not expect them to have the same sense of obligation about patient privacy that we do.

Cases reported in the press make excellent discussion guides for training. When Arthur Ashe disclosed his illness to the public, it was because his medical information had been leaked to the press and was about to be published. The public expressed sympathy for the heartache caused to Ashe and his family and outrage that someone in the medical profession could be so callous. Later cases publicized in the media included those of a state public health employee in Florida who allegedly passed a list of AIDS patients around a gay bar; the employee who sent Tammy Wynette's computerized medical records to a national tabloid; and the computer hacker who located Senator Robert Dole's medical records.

Exhibit 18.2. Sample Confidentiality and Conflict of Interest Agreement.

I hereby acknowledge, by my signature below, that I understand that the patient medical and financial information, records, and data to which I have knowledge and access in the course of my employment with the _____ (group name) is to be kept confidential, and this confidentiality is a term and condition of my employment. This information and any and all other information of a confidential nature shall not be disclosed to anyone under any circumstances, except to the extent necessary to fulfill my job requirements. The approval of my supervisor, administrator, or managing partner must first be obtained before any disclosure is made.

I hereby agree to avoid any activity that results in a real or apparent conflict of interest. I will not accept any fee or payment from anyone seeking to do business with the _____ (group name). I will not take advantage of any business opportunity learned of at work, and I will not use confidential information for personal gain under any circumstances whatsoever.

I understand and agree that any violation of this Agreement is grounds for disciplinary action, up to and including discharge.

_____   _____
Signature of Employee   Date

                                        _____
                                         Annual Review Date

Source: Connecticut Medical Insurance Company. Reprinted with permission.

Disclosure of information without authorization can create significant financial loss for an organization. St. Clare's Hospital and Health Center in New York was sued for $10 million when hospital records of a congresswoman were allegedly leaked to the press (Gorman, 1996). In a Connecticut case, a woman told her physician that she had tested HIV-positive. A medical assistant in the practice had two sons who were acquaintances of the patient, and as reported in *American Medical News* ("Decision Protects AIDS Patient Privacy," 1996, p. 24), the assistant "disclosed the information to her sons, who apparently told other people also. Then Jane Doe's children learned of their mother's illness from their friends." A settlement was reached in the patient's suit against the medical assistant.

In a Florida case, a hospital medical records employee was visited at work by her teenage daughter. As a prank, the employee's daughter called former emergency department patients, telling them that their tests indicated that they were HIV-positive. When she told a teenager that her lab tests were positive for HIV and pregnancy, that young woman attempted suicide. The employee's daughter was charged as an adult and received five years probation (McKenzie, 1996).

Visual reminders are a helpful tool in ongoing education. At the University of Connecticut Health Center in Farmington, a sign posted in each elevator reads, "Visitors and staff are reminded of the patient's right to privacy and the confidential nature of medical information."

Another visual reminder is the confidentiality statement on a fax cover sheet. Here is a sample statement: "Unauthorized interception of this telephonic communication is a violation of federal and state law. The documents accompanying this fax transmission may contain confidential information that is legally privileged, and the information provided is intended only for the use of the recipient. Any unauthorized release of information is strictly prohibited. If you have received this fax in error, please notify the sender by telephone and destroy this information. Thank you."

See that your vendors have a strong commitment to protecting patient confidentiality. Include confidentiality provisions in contracts with dictation, answering, collection, information management, and other services. Require them to have their employees and representatives sign confidentiality agreements. If services are performed off-site, what procedures does the vendor have in place to transport, process, and secure patient information? Ask computer vendors about systems that require a fingerprint instead of simply a password. Do not provide patient diagnoses to collection agencies. If your hospital is holding a program on patient confidentiality, ask whether you can invite your vendors to attend. Or request that the program be videotaped and circulate the tape to your vendors for viewing.

Consider using envelopes that list only your address, not your practice name. Some psychiatric practices tell patients that members of the practice will not acknowledge them in public unless the patient speaks to them first.

Patients have the right to expect that their medical information will be protected and not be divulged, except as required by law, without their permission. To be lax about protecting patient confidentiality can destroy one and possibly all of your relationships with patients.

Let Patients Know That You Understand How They Feel

In his book *Come as You Are*, Rev. G. Peter Fleck (1993, p. 18) retells his daughter's story about an airplane trip she took at the age of thirteen. "She was afraid and kept watching one of the engines from her window seat, as if her watching the engine would reduce, if not eliminate, the danger of malfunction. When lunch was served she did not eat. Whereupon her neighbor, a middle-aged gentleman who had finished his lunch, said to her, 'You can eat your lunch, kiddo. I'll watch the engine for you.'"

That's empathy. Empathy is being able to feel a situation as another person feels it. A patient may perceive empathy in an appropriate touch, especially when you hold a patient's hand or touch the patient where he hurts. Conversation helps to develop empathy, for it is in conversation that people discover shared experiences and feelings. One dermatologist, with his practice manager's permission, tells patients about the manager's experience, seven years before, with malignant melanoma.

Use words that are familiar to your patient. If your patient uses the word *terrific* and you say, "I think you are doing a terrific job with your insulin," you have communicated in a subtle but meaningful way that you have something in common with your patient.

Be a Resource for Your Patients

Companies like to talk about value these days. In boardrooms across America, the same question is asked over and over again: "What are we doing to provide more value for our customers?" We perceive value when an organization does something that other companies don't do. The men from my window-cleaning service take their shoes off when they enter my house. No other cleaning service has

> We perceive value when an organization does something that other companies don't do.

ever done that, and if I changed services, I think the new window washers would view me as crazy if I suggested it. It's the something extra that creates value and therefore loyalty.

One physician learned an important strategy for creating value from his accountant. Each year, the accountant sent him a free report showing the physician's financial status compared to prior years. The reports showed cumulative information that the physician felt he wouldn't get if he ever decided to change accountants. The report was of such value to him that he began to provide a similar free service to his patients. After each routine physical examination, patients receive a cumulative health report. Patients find the report very persuasive in motivating them to adopt healthier behaviors.

Contributing to the success of your patient's business is another strategy that can develop loyalty. If you are in a position to refer a customer or client to a patient, ask the patient first. "From time to time, people ask me about the services of a good dry cleaner. I'd like to be able to say that one of my patients is in the business and could help them. Would that be helpful to you?" Do not create unrealistic expectations. Offer only what you can deliver. Alert your staff to this strategy as well. Helping them adopt the habit of making referrals can ultimately result in more referrals for your practice.

Knowing what patients need before they need it and offering assistance at the appropriate time also creates value. For example, when you bought your first VCR, you might have lived with the blinking 12:00 for some time before figuring out how to program it. Suppose, though, that the person who sold you the VCR called you a few days later to see how it was working and offered to walk you through setting the time. What would your perception be of that salesperson?

The *Wall Street Journal* ran a feature story on Alan Brunacini, fire chief for the city of Phoenix, Arizona (Petzinger, 1997). His firefighters are prepared to meet the needs that some victims will have after a fire. They are ready to assist business owners with finding emergency office space and alternate telephone service. Paramedics will contact relatives and secure an accident victim's home if necessary. A child whose home has been involved in a fire receives a teddy bear. The chief advises his firefighters not to impose their values on others but instead to find out what is most important to the victims. If the business owner wants to save a hard drive instead of a filing cabinet, firefighters respect his decision. Good Samaritans are thanked and not pushed aside when firefighters arrive. The result? By being prepared to provide what people need, the fire department is viewed favorably by those who fund its salary and equipment budgets. Chief Brunacini said it best: "When you are confused, beat up and hurting, nothing feels as good as some calm, capable, credible, concerned person paying attention" (p. B1).

Your knowledge of your patient, combined with your knowledge of the patient's medical condition, means that you often know what your patient will need even before he does. Taking advantage of your expertise to prepare to meet those needs will encourage your patient's loyalty.

Act Consistently to Help Patients Know What to Expect

Consistent behavior encourages your patient to trust you and enhances your credibility. If you are engaging and sociable during one appointment and distracted and abrupt during another, the patient suffers the anxiety of not knowing what to expect. Credibility and trust are closely linked. The root origin of the word *credibility* is *credo,* meaning "I trust or believe." When you treat patients inconsistently, you lose credibility in the process. When you lose credibility, patients have a more difficult time trusting you.

When my husband and I were taking our son, Thomas, to see Peter Hughes, an orthopedic surgeon, Dr. Hughes was consistently calm and cheerful every time he saw Thomas, despite the filled reception area and the hectic pace at the reception desk in his practice. He never seemed harried, and he made Thomas feel that he had all the time in the world for him. He reduced our anxiety about Thomas's condition because we could count on him to meet our expectations every time.

Let Your Patient Know What Will Happen Next

Be clear about who will do what next. If you say, "Your test results will be back in a week," you leave the patient wondering whether you will call him or he should call you. Be specific about what you will do after visits and what your patient should do.

When you are letting your patient know what will happen next, weave "for you" into your explanation. This strategy is an easy habit to develop, after a bit of practice. "I'll be happy to schedule the next visit for you." "Let me put the lead apron on for you." "I think we should do this test for you first." The use of "for you" subtly but effectively reminds the patient that he is your focus and priority.

Be Responsive

If you want loyal patients, be responsive to them. Loyalty may come more naturally to some patients than to others, but loyalty is really the result of what you do to earn the patient's trust. A sense of trust must be the foundation for a loyal relationship.

Be accessible for urgent needs. You can trust someone when you know she will be there for you when you really need her. Actions that foster trust include seeing patients who are in pain the same day, calling patients personally with test results, and taking time to review all medications a patient is taking. Returning telephone calls when promised also increases a patient's trust in you.

Lou Holtz, the former Notre Dame coach, has said that in every relationship, people have three questions: "First, can I trust you? Second, are you committed to excellence? Third, will you care about me?" Think of the most positive relationships you have had as a patient and see if you can draw on those positive memories to identify strategies that will be meaningful and memorable for your patients.

Find Something in Common with Your Patient

You must establish an emotional bond with your patient for him to be happy about returning to see you. You can often create emotional links by discovering what you have in common with another person. As a freshman in college, you were probably repeatedly asked, "What's your major?" Some hotels include the employee's hometown on name badges, knowing that being from the same area can create connections between people. People often look for such connections as a relationship begins. When President Reagan was being prepared for surgery after being shot, he said to the surgeon, "I hope you're a Republican." The surgeon answered with this reassuring and touching statement: "Mr. President, today we're all Republicans."

Sophisticated patients understand that "a physician with a similar life experience may prove more compassionate and more willing to develop a lasting friendship" (Garb, 1992, p. 22). Beginning in the seventies, more female patients began to prefer being seen by female physicians; some patients today seek out physicians of the same race, ethnic group, religion, and sexual orientation. One patient in a metropolitan area was determined to locate an obstetrician who was pregnant with her first child—and found her!

People like people who like them. Have you ever said to yourself, "Why can't my patient be more like me?" In trying to find something in common, talk to your patient about the subject he is most interested in—that is, himself. And remember, the one thing that you can have in common with every patient is his best interest.

Let Patients Know That You Appreciate Them

Many patients are grateful for the care, cure, or comfort they receive from their physicians and other members of the health care team. Their gratitude may be expressed in a variety of ways: a verbal or written thank-you, a holiday card or gift, or perhaps follow-through on your recommendations. Keep all personal correspondence you receive from patients. A thank-you note, gift card, holiday card, or postcard often contains personal information that can be a quick cue for discussion with your patient during your next consultation. How often do you thank patients for choosing you and entrusting you with their health and lives?

People stay where they are appreciated. Say thank you often. "Thank you for waiting." "Thank you for the holiday card." "Thank you for completing the patient satisfaction survey. We are considering your suggestion." When you praise a patient, be brief, specific, and of course, sincere. If you can't think of something specific to comment on, a sincere, "Thanks for coming to see me," or, "I enjoy having you as a patient," is still meaningful.

Your patient knows that he is not your only patient. But wouldn't it be nice if every patient felt as though he was your favorite patient? If you can't generate that much enthusiasm, make an effort to find a reason to be happy to see your patient. *Reflexive self-concept* is a term used to describe the patient's perception of what the doctor thinks of him as a person. Reflexive self-concept is a predictor of patient satisfaction and compliance (Ellig, Whittemore, and Green, 1960). One patient, describing her feelings of loyalty for her physician, said, "No matter what happened, and I had a lot there for awhile, she was always happy to see me, happy to help me."

People often give gifts to express appreciation to others. Dentists have traditionally given toothbrushes, but in medicine, all too often the "gift" is a supply of drug samples. Drug samples are a poor substitute for your time and attention. The amount of time patients think they need varies dramatically from one patient to the next. One patient expects an hour of your time, another is impatiently tapping her fingers after ten minutes. Give your patient undivided attention for the first sixty seconds of your meeting. It is not always easy to do this, as telephones are ringing and others in the practice need you "for just a second." However, when you can do it, you will create the impression that you have spent a meaningful amount of time with the patient.

One physician noticed that her patients often began conversations with her by saying, "I'm sorry to bother you, I know how busy you are . . ." This kind of statement was a cue to her that she might appear to be rushed when she spoke with patients. She formed a habit of pausing before responding to a patient's apologetic statement. After the pause, she would begin her response with, "Mr. Jefferson, I'm never too busy for you," in a kind, upbeat tone of voice.

Mark Twain said, "I could live six months on a compliment." Is there a greater compliment than conveying to someone through sincere listening that what he has to say is important? Could your patient participate in an inservice education program with you?

Could he be featured in your organization's newsletter? Could he lead a support group?

Stay in Touch

Staying in touch with patients between visits is another way to build loyal relationships. Sending a bill is not what I mean. If all a patient ever receives from you is a bill, he may feel that the only time he hears from you is when you want something from him. Begin the process of staying in touch by mentioning your next meeting while your patient is still in the office. Say something about the next time you expect to be in contact, or schedule needed routine tests. This strategy can be used even if you don't expect to see your patient again. Dr. Reuben Wekselman of Burlingame, California, treated a nine-year-old boy whose arm was broken while he was on vacation in the area. He concluded the visit by asking the boy's mother, "Would you drop me a card and tell me how he makes out?" The mother mentioned Wekselman's thoughtfulness to all of the friends she saw in California and to many people back home in Massachusetts too.

A letter and a consultation have greater value for a patient than a consultation alone. A New York City physician dictates his consultation findings and has his dictation service prepare his notes in the form of a letter to his patients. All the patients in the practice tell him how much they enjoy receiving the letters. Many patients keep them.

Follow-up telephone calls can benefit almost every patient and are very well received. A call to ask how a medication is working or how a visit to a specialist turned out is long remembered. Dr. K. J. Lee of New Haven, Connecticut, calls patients even if he is out of state on business. His patients are very pleased when he takes the time to call them from Chicago or San Francisco or wherever he happens to be (K. J. Lee, personal interview with the author, 1997).

If a large number of your patients spend time in other parts of the country, consider having a toll-free number for them to contact you. The monthly expense will be small, and the degree of satisfaction with it will be high, because it's so unexpected.

A personal note from you or any member of the practice will exceed your patient's expectations every time. Invest in a supply of note cards and encourage employees to send handwritten notes whenever they think of it. Many people have difficulty putting a short note on a long page of stationery, and thus good intentions get lost because people do not have enough to say or enough time to fill up the entire page; note cards are the perfect solution. A short note can be as simple as this: "Thank you for being so understanding about the problem you experienced. If I can help you in the future, my card is enclosed." Most people, in sorting their mail, give handwritten correspondence special attention.

A newsletter, announcement of a health program, subscription to a health magazine, birthday card, or cassette tape of information are other methods of staying in touch between visits. If you send holiday or birthday cards to patients, sign them more personally than "XYZ Clinic." Ask everyone in the practice to sign the card or ask the patient's primary caregiver to write a personal note. Some consultants suggest sending a Thanksgiving or New Year's card rather than a Christmas or Hanukkah card. Your note might read, "I'm wishing you and your family a New Year with much happiness. Remember, I'm always happy to serve you."

Consistency-Flexibility Model

To manage patient expectations in a way that makes those expectations positive yet realistic, you have to achieve a balance of consistency and flexibility: consistency so that patients know what to expect, flexibility so that patients feel that you identify and respect their unique preferences. Standardize routine functions as much as possible. When you have many different ways to do things, those things take more time to accomplish. Consistency doesn't mean that you never change anything; it means that you make adjustments and improvements when needed but always with the knowledge of those who need to know—including patients.

It would be impossible for a practice to adopt all the strategies identified in this book. If you choose just ten strategies, with the goal of balancing service consistency and flexibility, you should be able to implement those strategies successfully. The list that follows is my suggested top ten. You might adopt some or all of these or substitute some of your own. If every member of your practice follows your ten strategies every day, your organization will become known for providing exceptional patient care.

1. We acknowledge patients when they arrive. We say hello first.

2. We answer telephone calls within three rings with a consistent greeting.

3. We use the patient's name at least once during each conversation.

4. We take a moment to observe the patient's communication style and respond in a manner that will make the patient feel comfortable.

5. We remember to explain to patients what is going to happen next.

6. We listen to patients without interrupting them.

7. We watch for verbal and nonverbal signs that the patient is not satisfied or is concerned about something. We are proactive in identifying and responding to problems.

8. We respect patient confidentiality at all times. We do not divulge who our patients are, even to members of our own families.

9. We do what we say we will do, when we say we will do it.

10. When a patient is leaving, we say good-bye warmly and wish him well or say we look forward to seeing him again.

◆ ◆ ◆ ◆ ◆ ◆ ◆

Why are some people memorable in our lives, while others become names and faces we never recall? As a physician, you can create experiences and relationships that change people's lives forever.

Patients expect that their physicians will have integrity. Your integrity depends on maintaining the confidentiality of patient information, telling the truth, doing what you say you will do, accepting responsibility when something goes wrong, and respecting every person.

You earn money not for your knowledge but for what you do with your knowledge. It's not what you know, but what you do with what you know that counts. Time constraints prevent most people from paying attention to the simple things that make a difference. Challenge yourself to be extraordinary! Gain a return on the investment of your time spent reading this book by implementing some of the strategies in your practice. Your patients will be happier, and so will you. And being cared for by a physician who loves what she does may be the greatest patient satisfier of all.

> **It's not what you know, but what you do with what you know that counts.**

Patients want flexibility, responsiveness, consistency, and quality in their relationship with you. Regardless of the clinical outcome, patients will perceive quality when they receive interest, understanding, empathy, and compassion. Patients need to feel that they are safe and secure, that they belong and are important. By identifying what your patient needs and respecting what he wants, you exceed your patient's expectations and are the memorable physician you intended to be when you entered the profession.

References

"Alabama Hospital's ER Access Program Had Short Life." *Modern Healthcare*,
June 24, 1996, p. 72.

Alexander, R. "Metropolitan Diary." *New York Times*, May 7, 1997, p. C2. Copyright © 1996/97 by The New York Times Co. Reprinted by permission.

Anderson, E. "Physician Won Malpractice Case, But Still Lost a Lot." *American Medical News*, Mar. 4, 1996, pp. 15–16.

Anton, J. "Customer Relationship Management." Presentation at the *Inc.* Customer Service Strategies Conference, San Diego, Calif., Mar. 1996.

Appleby, C. "Time Is on Their Side." *Hospitals and Health Networks*, Oct. 20, 1996a, pp. 49–50.

Appleby, C. "Timeliness Is Next to Godliness." *Hospitals and Health Networks*, Aug. 5, 1996b, p. 40.

Atkins, C. "Before Battle: Thoughts on Doctor-Patient Relationship." *American Medical News*, May 5, 1997, p. 29.

Bannon, L. "Plastic Surgeons Are Told to Pay More Attention to Appearances." *Wall Street Journal*, Feb. 4, 1997, p. B1.

Barsky, A. J. "Hidden Reasons Some Patients Visit Doctors." *Annals of Internal Medicine*, 1981, *94*(4), 492–498.

Barsky, J. D. *World Class Customer Satisfaction*. Burr Ridge, Ill.: Irwin, 1995.

Beatty, S. "Ad Man Felt He'd Deserved Break Since 1981." *Wall Street Journal*, July 31, 1997, pp. B11–B12.

Beckman, H. B., Markakis, K. M., Suchman, A. L., and Frankel, R. M. "The Doctor-Patient Relationship and Malpractice." *Archives of Internal Medicine*, 1994, *154*(12), 1365–1370.

Benson, H., and Friedman, R. "Harnessing the Power of the Placebo Effect and Renaming It 'Remembered Wellness.'" *Annual Review of Medicine*, 1996, *47*, 193–199.

Berglas, S. "Liar, Liar, Pants on Fire." *Inc.*, Aug. 1997, p. 33. Reprinted with permission of *Inc.* magazine, Goldhirsh Group, Inc., 38 Commercial Wharf, Boston, Ma. 02110. *Liar, liar, pants on fire*, Steven Berglas, August 1997. (http://www.inc.com). Reproduced by permission of the publisher via Copyright Clearance Center, Inc.

Bethune, G. "Listening to You." *Profiles*, June 1995, p. 8.

Binkley, C. "Harrah's Builds Database About Patrons." *Wall Street Journal*, Sept. 2, 1997, p. B9.

Blueprints for Service Quality: The Federal Express Approach. (2nd ed.) New York: American Management Association Briefing, 1994.

Bowles, J., and Hammond, J. *Beyond Quality.* New York: Putnam, 1991.

Bryant, P., and Underwood, J. *Bear: The Hard Life and Good Times of Alabama's Coach Bryant.* Boston: Little, Brown, 1974.

Buchanan, K., and others. "Patients' Beliefs About Cancer Management." *Supportive Care in Cancer*, 1996, 4(2), 110–117.

Bursztajn, H. J. "Substituting Alliance for Alienation: Supporting the Human Side in Changing Health Care." Paper presented at the New England Healthcare Assembly, Falmouth, Mass., July 1997.

Bursztajn, H. J., and Brodsky, A. "A New Resource for Managing Malpractice Risks in Managed Care." *Archives of Internal Medicine*, 1996, 156, 2057–2063.

Cafferky, M. *Patients Build Your Practice: Word of Mouth Marketing for Healthcare Practitioners.* New York: McGraw-Hill, 1994.

Caggiano, C. "How Do I Improve Our Customer Service?" *Inc.*, Aug. 1997, p. 92.

Calkins, D., and others. "Patient-Physician Communication at Hospital Discharge and Patients' Understanding of the Postdischarge Treatment Plan." *Archives of Internal Medicine*, 1997, 157, 1026–1030.

Cantoni, C. J. "The Consulting Mystique." *Wall Street Journal*, Mar. 10, 1997, p. A18.

Carlzon, J. *Moments of Truth.* New York: HarperCollins, 1987.

Carlzon, J. "The Moment of Truth." Presentation at the *Inc.* Customer Service Strategies Conference, San Diego, Calif., Mar. 1996.

Carman, D., and Britten, N. "Confidentiality of Medical Records: The Patient's Perspective." *British Journal of General Practice*, 1995, 45(398), 485–488.

Cecil, D. W., and Killeen, I. "Control, Compliance and Satisfaction in the Family Practice Encounter." *Family Medicine*, 1997, 29(9), 653–657.

Champy, J. "Business 101, the Hard Way." *New York Times*, Aug. 16, 1997.

Chase, M. "Not All Star Doctors Are Going to Shine in Giving Patient Care." *Wall Street Journal*, Sept. 23, 1996, p. B1.

Clifford, R. *Only When I Laugh*. London: Warner Books, 1982.

Cohen, S. L. "Should Health Care Come with a Warranty?" *New York Times*, Nov. 10, 1996, p. 12.

Coley, C. M., and others. "Preferences for Home vs. Hospital Care Among Low-Risk Patients with Community-Acquired Pneumonia." *Archives of Internal Medicine*, 1996, *156*(14), 1565–1571.

"Complaint Puts to Rest Maternity Room Lullaby." *Boston Globe*, Mar. 18, 1997, p. B11.

Connellan, T. K., and Zemke, R. *Sustaining Knock Your Socks Off Service*. New York: AMACOM, 1993.

Conner, D. R. *Managing at the Speed of Change*. New York: Random House, 1992.

Covey, S. R. *The Seven Habits of Highly Effective People*. New York: Simon & Schuster, 1989.

Dansky, K., and Miles, J. "Patient Satisfaction with Ambulatory Healthcare Services: Waiting Time and Filling Time." *Hospital and Health Services Administration*, 1997, *42*(2), 165–177.

Davidhizer, R. "What's in a Name?" *Advance for Nurse Practitioners*, Dec. 1995, p. 58.

Davidow, W. H., and Uttal, B. *Total Customer Service*. New York: HarperCollins, 1989.

"Decision Protects AIDS Patient Privacy." *American Medical News*, May 20, 1996, p. 24.

Delbanco, T. "Enriching the Doctor-Patient Relationship by Inviting the Patient's Perspective." *Annals of Internal Medicine*, 1992, *116*(5), 414.

Dewar, A. L., and Morse, J. M. "Unbearable Incidents: Failure to Endure the Experience of Illness." *Journal of Advanced Nursing*, 1995, *22*(5), 957–964.

"The Disney Approach to Quality Service." Presentation and handout at Disney Co. conference on customer service, Orlando, Fla., 1996.

"Doc, Can't You Give Me a Few More Weeks Off?" *Business & Health*, Sept. 1995, p. 11.

Drucker, S. "Who Is the Best Restaurateur in America?" *New York Times Magazine*, Mar. 10, 1996, pp. 45–47, 104.

Eisenberg, D. M. "Advising Patients Who Seek Alternative Medical Therapies." *Annals of Internal Medicine*, 1997, *127*(1), 61–69.

Ellig, R., Whittemore, R., and Green, M. "Patient Participation in a Pediatric Program." *Journal of Health and Human Behavior*, 1960, *1*, 183.

"Empathy Beats Fancy Food in Assuring Patient Satisfaction." *Health Measures*, Mar. 1997, p. 11.

Epstein, H. "Technology Redux." *Inc. Technology*, 1997, *1*, 27.

Eracker, S. A., Kirscht, J. P., and Becker, M. H. "Understanding and Improving Patient Compliance." *Annals of Internal Medicine*, 1984, *100*, 258–268.

Eye on Patients: A Report from the American Hospital Association and the Picker Institute. Chicago: American Hospital Association, 1996.

Fabricant, F. "Going Beyond 'Hi, My Name Is Pat.'" *New York Times*, Sept. 4, 1996, pp. C1, C3.

Fink, M. "Insider." *People*, July 22, 1996, p. 28.

Finlay, P. M., Atkinson, J. M., and Moos, K. F. "Orthognathic Surgery: Patient Expectations; Psychological Profile and Satisfaction with Outcome." *British Journal of Oral & Maxillofacial Surgery*, 1995, *33*(1), 9–14.

Fitzpatrick, J. "The Writer: Bringing a Story to Life." *New York Times*, Apr. 6, 1997, Connecticut sec., pp. 1, 13.

Fleck, G. P. *Come as You Are.* Boston: Beacon Press, 1993.

Ford, L. "Customers as Partners: How to Build Loyalty and Repeat Business." Presentation at the *Inc.* Customer Service Strategies Conference, San Diego, Calif., Mar. 1996.

Foss, K. R., and Tenholder, M. F. "Expectations and Needs of Persons with Family Members in an Intensive Care Unit as Opposed to a General Ward." *Southern Medical Journal*, 1993, 86(4), 380–384.

Froelich, G. W., and Welch, H. G. "Meeting Walk-In Patients' Expectations for Testing: Effects on Satisfaction." *Journal of General Internal Medicine*, 1996, *11*(8), 470–474.

Fromm, B., and Schlesinger, L. *The Real Heroes of Business.* New York: Doubleday, 1993.

Garb, M. "Like Doctor, Like Patient." *American Medical News*, Sept. 14, 1992, pp. 22–24.

"Gas Station Offers Mammograms." *American Medical News*, Sept. 2, 1996, p. 9.

Gentry, C. "HMOs' Cost-Cutting Frenzy Is a Pain." *Boston Globe*, July 4, 1995, p. 12.

Gianelli, D. M. "Fertility Clinic: Baby in Three Tries or Your Money Back." *American Medical News*, Sept. 25, 1995, p. 4.

Goldsmith, M. "Retaining High Impact Performers." *Leader to Leader*, 1996, *1*(1), 6–8.

Gore, A. *The Best Kept Secrets in Government.* New York: Random House, 1996.

Gorman, C. "Who's Looking at Your Files?" *Time*, May 6, 1996, pp. 60–62.

Gruner, S. "Hands on Marketing." *Inc.*, Aug. 1997, p. 93.

Gutheil, T. G., Bursztajn, H. J., and Brodsky, A. "Malpractice Prevention Through the Sharing of Uncertainty." *New England Journal of Medicine*, 1984, *311*(1), 49–51.

Hall, J. A., Roter, D. L., Milburn, M. A., and Daltroy, L. H. "Patients' Health as a Predictor of Physician and Patient Behavior in Medical Visits." *Medical Care*, 1996, *34*(12), 1205–1218.

Harmetz, A. "Master Joker Who Never Forgets." *New York Times*, Sept. 28, 1989, pp. C1, C18.

Harper, M. B., and Wisian, N. B. "Care of Bereaved Parents: A Study of Patient Satisfaction." *Journal of Reproductive Medicine*, 1994, *39*(2), 80–86.

Hart, C. *Extraordinary Guarantees: A New Way to Build Quality Throughout Your Company and Ensure Satisfaction for Your Customers*. New York: AMA-COM, 1993.

Hawken, P. A. *Growing a Business*. New York: Simon & Schuster, 1987.

Hays, M. "Passwords Aren't Enough." *Healthcare Informatics*, Apr. 1997, p. 102.

Heskett, J. L., and others. "Putting the Service-Profit Chain to Work." *Harvard Business Review*, Mar.–Apr. 1994, pp. 164–174.

Hilts, E. "Restaurant Review." *Fairfield Advocate*, Apr. 1996, p. 15.

Hofman, M. "What's in Store for Mobil? Check Your Local 5 & 10." *Inc.*, Feb. 1997, p. 18.

Holmes, O. W., Sr. *The Professor at the Breakfast Table*. 1860.

Holzer, J. F. "A New Approach to Informed Consent Can Reduce Claims." *Pediatric Annals*, 1991, *20*(2), 64–68.

Hopkins, T. *How to Master the Art of Selling*. New York: Warner Books, 1982.

"Hospital Stands Behind Promise of Fast Service." *Modern Healthcare*, Aug. 21, 1995, pp. 148–149.

Jeffrey, N. "Hospitals Use TV Spots to Boost Business." *Wall Street Journal*, Sept. 26, 1996, p. B10.

Johnson, J. A., and King, K. B. "Influence of Expectations About Symptoms on Delay in Seeking Treatment During Myocardial Infarction." *American Journal of Critical Care*, 1995, *4*(1), 29–35.

Kaiser Family Foundation and Agency for Healthcare Policy and Research study. *Americans as Healthcare Consumers: The Role of Quality Information. A National Survey*. Palo Alto, Calif.: Henry J. Kaiser Family Foundation, Oct. 1996.

Kaplan, S. H., and others. "Patient and Visit Characteristics Related to Physicians' Participatory Decision-Making Style." *Medical Care*, 1995, *33*(12), 1176–1187.

Katon, W., and others. "Collaborative Management to Achieve Depression Treatment Guidelines." *Journal of Clinical Psychiatry*, 1997, *58*(Suppl. 1), 20–23.

Kelliher, M. "Service Guarantees in Health Care," Presentation at the New England Healthcare Assembly Meeting, Boston, Mar. 1997.

Keyes, C., and Augello, T. "Teaching Residents and Medical Students to Disclose Mistakes." *Forum*, 1997, *18*(1), 6–7.

Kravitz, R. L., and others. "Prevalence and Source of Patients' Unmet Expectations for Care." *Annals of Internal Medicine*, 1996, *125*(9), 770–771.

Langreth, R. "Doctor, Doctor." *Wall Street Journal*, Oct. 24, 1997, p. R4. Reprinted by permission of *Wall Street Journal*, © 1997 Dow Jones & Company, Inc. All rights reserved worldwide.

Leedham, B., Meyerowitz, B. E., Muirhead, J., and Frist, W. H. "Positive Expectations Predict Health After Heart Transplant." *Health Psychology*, 1995, *14*(1), 74–79.

Lenzner, R., and Johnson, S. "Peter Drucker—Still the Youngest of Minds." *Forbes*, Mar. 10, 1997, p. 125.

Levinson, W., and others. "Patient-Physician Communication: The Relationship with Malpractice Claims Among Primary Care Physicians and Surgeons." *Journal of the American Medical Association*, 1997, *277*(7), 553–559.

Levitt, T. *The Marketing Imagination*. New York: Free Press, 1986.

Lieber, R. "Storytelling: A New Way to Get Close to Your Customers." *Fortune*, Feb. 3, 1997, pp. 102–108.

Ligos, M. "Express Meetings." *Successful Meetings*, May 1997, p. 18.

Linn, M. W., Linn, B. S., and Stein, S. R. "Satisfaction with Ambulatory Care and Compliance in Older Patients." *Medical Care*, 1982, *10*(6), 606–614.

Lippman, H. "Science and Sensibility." *Business & Health*, Mar. 1997, p. 6.

Llinas, J. L. "Hobson's Choice." *Medical Economics*, Feb. 4, 1991, p. 135.

MacStravic, R. S. "Using Marketing to Reduce Malpractice Costs in Health Care." *Health Care Management Review*, 1989, *14*(4), 51–56.

Mannello, T. *A CQI System for Healthcare*. New York: Quality Resources, 1995.

May, R. *The Meaning of Anxiety*. New York: Norton, 1977.

Maxa, R. "Portraits." *USAir Magazine*, Nov. 1996, p. 112.

McKenna, R. *Real Time: Preparing for the Age of the Never Satisfied Customer*. Boston: Harvard Business School Press, 1997.

McKenzie, D. "Banking on Security." *infoCARE*, May–June 1996, pp. 35–39.

Michaels, E. "Doctors Can Improve On Way They Deliver Bad News, MD Maintains." Interview with R. Buckman. *Canadian Medical Association Journal*, 1992, *146*(4), 564–566.

Millman, D. *Way of the Peaceful Warrior*. Tiburon, Calif.: Kramer, 1980.

Miranda, J., and Brody, R. V. "Communicating Bad News." *Western Journal of Medicine*, 1992, *156*, 83–85.

Montague, J. "Do as I Say, Not as I Don't." *Hospitals and Health Networks*, Mar. 5, 1995a, p. 47.

Montague, J. "Making Hospitals More Hospitable." *Hospitals and Health Networks*, Sept. 20, 1995b, p. 64.

Moore, S. M., and Kramer, F. M. "Women's and Men's Preferences for Cardiac Rehabilitation Features." *Journal of Cardiopulmonary Rehabilitation*, 1996, 16(3), 163–168.

Munthe, A. *The Story of San Michele*. London: John Murray, 1929.

Nedelman, P. Letter to the editor. *Patriot Ledger*, Apr. 25, 1996, p. 14.

Nelson, E. D., and Larson, C. "Patients' Good and Bad Surprises: How Do They Relate to Overall Patient Satisfaction?" *Quality Review Bulletin*, 1993, 19(3).

Nidecker, A. "Somatic Complaints Can Match Mood Disorders." *Family Practice News*, July 1, 1997, p. 53.

Oscar, G. "The Influence of Patient Expectations on Learning Experience." *Journal of the Canadian Association of Nephrology Nurses and Technicians*, Spring 1996, 6(2), 23–25.

"Outliers." *Modern Healthcare*, Nov. 4, 1996, p. 60.

Pereira, J. "A Small Toy Store Manages to Level the Playing Field." *Wall Street Journal*, Dec. 20, 1996, p. 1.

Peters, T. *The Pursuit of Wow*. New York: Random House, 1994.

Petkanas, C. "South of France, North of Heaven." *Travel and Leisure*, Mar. 1995, p. 119.

Petzinger, T., Jr. "Brunacini's Crew Puts Out Flames Then Puts Out Food for Fido." *Wall Street Journal*, Sept. 12, 1997, p. B1.

Pichert, J. W., and others. "Understanding the Etiology of Serious Medical Events Involving Children: Implications for Pediatricians and Their Risk Managers." *Pediatric Annals*, 1997, 26, 160–172.

Preston, J. "New HMO Rules Expand Patient Rights and Create an Arbitration Panel." *New York Times*, Feb. 5, 1997, p. B1.

Reichheld, F. F. *The Loyalty Effect*. Boston: Harvard Business School Press, 1996.

Richardson, L. *Stop Telling, Start Selling*. New York: McGraw-Hill, 1994.

Rosenfield, J. "Strange Bedfellows." *Across the Board.*" Oct. 1997, pp. 9–10.

The Rotarian, Aug. 1996, p. 56.

"St. Vincent Form on Funeral Choices Angers Patient." *Santa Fe New Mexican*, Jan. 21, 1996, p. 1.

Schaaf, D. *Keeping the Edge: Giving Customers the Service They Demand*. New York: NAL/Dutton, 1995.

Schneiderman, J. "The Upside Down Pyramid: How Ritz-Carlton Maintains Excellence." Presentation at the *Inc.* Customer Service Strategies Conference, San Diego, Calif., Mar. 1996.

"Seattle Goes au Naturel." *Hospitals and Health Networks*, Mar. 20, 1996, p. 82.

Serb, C. "If You Liked the Food, Press 1." *Hospitals and Health Networks*, Apr. 5, 1997, p. 99.

Sharpe, M., and others. "Why Do Doctors Find Some Patients Difficult to Help?" *Quarterly Journal of Medicine*, 1994, *87*(3), 187–193.

Shulkin, D. J., and Ferniany, I. W. "The Effect of Developing Patient Compendiums for Critical Pathways on Patient Satisfaction." *American Journal of Medical Quality*, 1996, *11*(1), 43–45.

Snow, C. "For Hemophilia Health CEO, Work Hits Home." *Modern Healthcare*, Sept. 23, 1996, pp. 73–74.

Stelovich, S. "Framework for Handling Adverse Events." *Forum*, 1997, *18*(1), 8–9.

Stevens, A. "Where the Boys, Girls, Teens, Couples, Tots and Washing-Machine Salesmen Are." *Wall Street Journal*, May 16, 1997, pp. B1, B6.

Stuart, M. R., and Lieberman, J. A., III. *The Fifteen Minute Hour: Applied Psychotherapy for the Primary Care Physician.* New York: Praeger, 1986. Used with permission.

"Studies Suggest Religious Activities Can Improve Health." *American Medical News*, Mar. 4, 1996, p. 31.

Stull, W. B., Lo, B., and Charles, G. "Do Patients Want to Participate in Medical Decision-Making?" *Journal of the American Medical Association*, 1984, *252*, 2990–2994.

Suchman, A. L., Markakis, K., Beckman, H. B., and Frankel, R. "A Model of Empathetic Communication in the Medical Interview." *Journal of the American Medical Association*, 1997, *277*(8), 678–682.

Thompson, J. "How California Pizza Kitchen Maintains a Culture of Super Service." Presentation at the *Inc.* Customer Service Strategies Conference, Orlando, Fla., Mar. 1997.

"Town Thanks Its Doctor After Decades of Healing." *New York Times*, Sept. 30, 1996, p. 12.

Turner, S. "Insights from Playing Patient." *Hospitals and Health Networks*, Nov. 20, 1995, p. 50.

Ubel, P., and others. "Elevator Talk: Observational Study of Inappropriate Comments in a Public Space." *American Journal of Medicine*, Aug. 1995, *99*, 190–194.

Uhlmann, R. F., Inui, T. S., and Carter, W. B. "Patient Requests and Expectations." *Medical Care*, 1984, *22*(7), 681–685.

Vetto, J. T., Dubois, P. M., and Vetto, I. P. "The Impact of Distribution of a Patient-Education Pamphlet in a Multidisciplinary Breast Clinic." *Journal of Cancer Education*, 1996, *11*(3), 148–152.

Waitley, D. *Empires of the Mind*. New York: Morrow, 1995.

Walton, S. *Sam Walton: Made in America*. New York: Bantam Books, 1993.

Watson, T., Jr. *Father, Son & Co*. New York: Bantam Books, 1990.

Weiser, C. R. "Championing the Customer." *Harvard Business Review*, Nov.–Dec. 1995, pp. 113–116.

Whiteley, R. C. *The Customer Driven Company*. Reading, Mass.: Addison-Wesley, 1991.

Williams, S., Weinman, J., Dale, J., and Newman, S. "Patient Expectations: What Do Primary Care Patients Want from the GP and How Far Does Meeting Expectations Affect Patient Satisfaction?" *Family Practice*, 1995, *12*(2), 193–201.

Witman, A., Park, D., and Hardin, S. "How Do Patients Want Physicians to Handle Mistakes? A Survey of Internal Medicine Patients in an Academic Setting." *Archives of Internal Medicine*, 1996, *156*, 2565–2569.

Zemke, R. "The Eight Essentials of Delivering Knock-Your-Socks-Off Service." Presentation at the *Inc.* Customer Service Strategies Conference, San Diego, Calif., Mar. 1996.

Index